Guerilla Gynecology

Guerilla Gynecology

Donna M. Bell, MD

Writers Club Press
San Jose New York Lincoln Shanghai

Guerilla Gynecology

Writers Club Press
an imprint of iUniverse.com, Inc.

For information address:
iUniverse.com, Inc.
5220 S 16th, Ste. 200
Lincoln, NE 68512
www.iuniverse.com

ISBN: 0-595-15156-6

Printed in the United States of America

Contents

List of Illustrations

Preface

Welcome to *Guerilla Gynecology*, a primer for the woman left dazed and confused in the wake of a "Hit-and-Run" gynecologist. Seriously though, and in all fairness to my gynecological colleagues, managed care leaves us little or no time to educate you. Dividing up the typical 15 to 20-minute gynecology visit, you are allowed 5 minutes to undress, 5 minutes for your exam and another 5 minutes to get dressed again.

With the 1 to 5 minutes that may or may not be left, your gynecologist has to compress and translate 8 or more years of medical education and specialty training into terms you will hopefully understand. Some offices try to supplement these rushed explanations by distributing reading materials or utilizing Nurse-Educators. For many of you however, this still is not enough.

But why are so many explanations needed anyway?

No, I am not trying to shirk my responsibilities and I am not trying to demean you by expecting you to know everything. But a lot of you think that STD's go away if you stop having sex or that bread gives you yeast! Even more of you are not aware that you are supposed to make ovarian cysts with each and every menstrual cycle!

We may have been liberated since the 1970's, but over my 16 years of practice as a New York City obstetrician-gynecologist I have come to the conclusion that a lot of basic knowledge is lacking. This is not necessarily your fault however, since sex is still taboo in our society and anything having to with it is still a deep, dark and shameful secret. Since gynecology is basically sex, it is sill a secret for a lot of you.

Well, it does not have to remain a secret.

Arm yourself with the power of knowledge and read Guerilla Gynecology! It goes over 21 basic gynecological topics that most of you will experience in a lifetime and provides the full explanations that I always wanted to give my patients, but could not find the time to do so.

Be warned, the first half of *Guerilla Gynecology* that deals with menstrual-related problems reads like a laborious textbook. These complicated topics defy brevity and, not wanting to lapse into the role of a "Hit-and-Run" gynecologist, I detailed them for you turn you into a gynecologist. Rest-assured this is not my intention. It is possible to get intentionally. While plodding through these chapters, you may think that I am trying to through them, but you will probably have to take several breaks to do so. Fortunately, the remainder of the book that deals with infections is easier to read.

Guerilla Gynecology has many repetitive sections, but this is also intentional. Since many of the 21 topics are related to one another I am simply trying to drum key concepts into your head.

Lastly, if it seems like *Guerilla Gynecology* is geared towards women with problems, *it is*. Obviously, distressed patients made the most impression on me, but this does not mean that the rest of you are excluded.

Self-criticisms aside, I am confident that each woman who reads *Guerilla Gynecology* will gain enough information to make her subsequent visits less stressful and more efficient.

Part I

Introductory Topics

1

Sex Organs

SEX ORGANS or your genitals are an appropriate beginning since Gynecology would not exist without them. They start to develop as early as 4 weeks while you are still in your mother's womb. Your sex organs are virtually complete 16 weeks later.

Most of you are familiar with the medical terms for your internal sex organs since they are directly involved in reproduction.

Most of you are not as familiar with the medical terms for your external ones, however. Although the clitoris and urethra are well known, the rest are usually referred to as, "my lips" or "down there".

Therefore, this first chapter provides you with the proper medical terms, descriptions and functions for both sets of sex organs as well as a diagram of them (in Figure 1.) at the end.

External sex organs include your:

1. **Vulva** or the outer skin area encompassing all of the organs below.
2. **Clitoris** or the knob-like structure that provides sexual pleasure above the opening where your urine emerges.
3. **Urethral meatus** or opening where your urine emerges.

4. **Urethra** or the inch-long tube from your urethral meatus to your bladder.
5. **Skene glands openings** or three barely visible slits located on both sides of your urethral meatus that are connected to tiny glands that produce lubricating mucus. If infected, these glands can become quite swollen and painful.
6. **Vaginal orifice** or the entrance to your birth canal.
7. **Hymenal ring remnant** or the circular tissue rim about an inch behind the vaginal orifice that is leftover from your previously intact hymen.
8. **Bartholin gland opening** or the single slit located on both lower sides of the vaginal orifice that is also connected to a larger mucus lubrication gland. Again, they can become quite swollen and painful when infected.
9. **Fourchette** or the lower rim of your vaginal orifice.
10. **Labia majora** or the large outer genital lips closest to your thighs.
11. **Labia minora** or the small inner genital lips covered with regular skin on the outside and pink shiny moist tissue on the inside.
12. **Vestibule** or the entire pink shiny moist area from your clitoris to your fourchette, one labia minora to another and the vagina from the orifice to the hymenal ring remnant.
13. **Anus** or the opening to your rectum.
14. **Perineum** or the outer skin between your fourchette and anus.
15. **Mons** or the triangular area of hairy skin above your clitoris.

Internal sex organs include your:

1. **Vagina** or the birth canal from your hymenal ring remnant to your cervix. Your rectum is below it and your urethra and bladder are above it.

2. **Cervix** or the lower inch of your uterus that connects with your vagina and opens up during labor. It consists of an inner canal or **endocervix** and outer surface or **ectocervix.**
3. **Uterus** or womb is the fist-sized triangular structure above your cervix. It consists of a **cavity lined by the endometrium or glands** that are the source of periods if there is no pregnancy and an **outer myometrium or muscle layer** that pushes out blood and/or a pregnancy. Your bladder is in front of it, your rectum is behind it and your small bowel is draped over the rest of it.
4. **Fallopian tubes** or the pink earthworm-sized structures that extend from the top of your uterus on both sides to each ovary where their delicate finger-like ends scoop up your egg after its release. This is also where your egg meets sperm.
5. **Ovaries** or gonads are white prune-sized organs located at the ends of both tubes that produce eggs and sex hormones from **cysts** or fluid-filled sacs.
6. **Adnexa** or the area containing a tube, ovary and broad ligament along each side of your uterus that is also draped by small bowel.
7. **Broad ligaments** or the triangular tissue support bands traveling from each side of your pelvic bone to each side of your uterus that also includes blood vessels, a tube and an ovary.
8. **Peritoneum** or the thin, stretchy, shiny, moist pink tissue that lines the pelvic and abdominal cavity, covers all of their internal organs and becomes exquisitely tender when inflamed and/or infected.

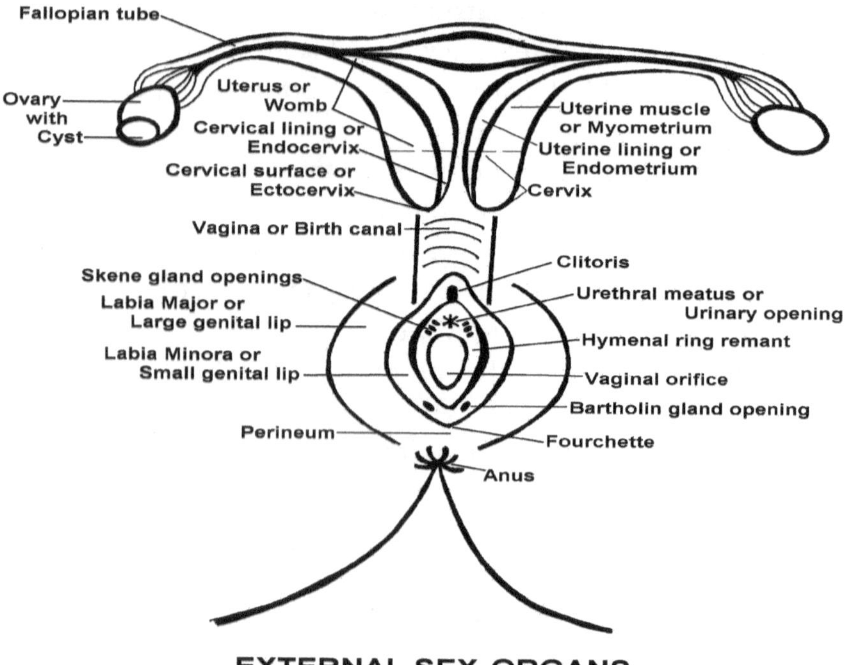
Figure 1.
INTERNAL SEX ORGANS
Fallopian tube
Ovary with Cyst
Uterus or Womb
Cervical lining or Endocervix
Cervical surface or Ectocervix
Uterine muscle or Myometrium
Uterine lining or Endometrium
Cervix
Vagina or Birth canal
Skene gland openings
Labia Major or Large genital lip
Labia Minora or Small genital lip
Perineum
Clitoris
Urethral meatus or Urinary opening
Hymenal ring remant
Vaginal orifice
Bartholin gland opening
Fourchette
Anus
EXTERNAL SEX ORGANS

2

Pelvic Exam

Since the pelvic exam is our main tool, trying to avoid one is not very realistic! Even if soft booties cover those barbaric stirrups and even if the speculum is kept nice and toasty, nobody likes being invaded, including myself. Unfortunately, this is not yet "Star Date Year 2124.5" when a blinking sensor can be waved externally over your torso to diagnose an internal problem!

There may be hoards of female gynecologists, but none of us have found a less intrusive way to evaluate our reproductive system. Our smaller fingers and female sensibility usually result in a more comfortable pelvic exam, however. So do as the British and "think of the Queen" when you are up in the rack with your bottom exposed!

EXAM PREPARATION

First of all, never douche before your pelvic exam! This washes away vaginal discharge, which is used to diagnose infection, as well as cervical cells that are needed for your PAP smear. Most importantly, douching never cleans you and actually gives you infections.

After arriving, please make a bathroom trip to empty your rectum and bladder. If you have are urinating a lot, pain when you urinate and/or lower abdominal pain however, please obtain clean wipes and a sterile container from the staff so your urine can be properly collected for later testing.

If you are bleeding, ask the staff for a pad before removing your tampon. Yes, you can have a pelvic exam in the midst of bleeding and I prefer to examine you then if you report heavy and/or irregular bleeding.

Several routine tests cannot be analyzed if you are bleeding, however so you may want to re-schedule if you need these.

In the exam room, take off your bra, pants, pantyhose and panties then put the gown on with the opening in the front so your breasts can be easily examined.

I am sorry if the instructions above sound obvious, but you would not believe how many women get up on the exam table with full bladders and their underwear still on!

VISUAL INSPECTION

VISUAL INSPECTION is the first part of your pelvic exam. This is a simple check of your clitoris, labia majora, perineum and anus for any growths, swelling, color and texture changes. Next, your labia minora are separated with two spread fingers in order to get a better view of your urethral meatus, vaginal orifice and other areas of your vestibule.

You should get into the habit of checking your own external sex organs. You will need a bright light that flexible and portable as well as a magnified mirror that supports itself. Get comfortable on your bed or hike one leg up on the toilet or bathroom counter, position both in between your legs and get acquainted with your body!

SPECULUM INSPECTION

SPECULUM INSPECTION is the second part of your pelvic exam. The speculum is the dreaded instrument that looks like a duck's bill attached to a handle and lever. When you press the lever, the each blade of the duck's bill separates to raise your vaginal roof and lower your vaginal floor.

Now, your vagina and cervix can be seen prior to sampling the latter for a PAP, GONORRHEA and CHLAMYDIA tests. The PAP looks for changes that occur before cervical cancer develops or actual cervical cancer itself. Gonorrhea and Chlamydia are infections passed from person-to person during sex that generally result in pain and make it hard for you to get pregnant in the future. All three have their own chapters in the last section of the book.

After the speculum is removed, a microscopic SALINE PREP TEST can be done in the office using a tiny bit of discharge from the top blade. The saline prep looks for vaginal infections and is discussed in more detail in the Yeast Chapter.

Bleeding prevents PAP, Gonorrhea and Chlamydia DNA-Probe and saline prep testing, though Gonorrhea and Chlamydia cultures can be sent if either is suspected.

Most speculums are plastic and disposable, though not technically sterile.

Metal speculums can be sterilized so they are ideal for surgical procedures. Since they are stronger, metal speculums are also used when your uterus is heavy as a result of pregnancy and/or fibroids (see this chapter), when more support is needed to separate the vaginal walls of heavy women or when you push a plastic one out! They get cold easily so warm water or a heating pad is often used to warm them.

Both come in different widths and lengths to accommodate all types of vaginas.

The speculum exam can be quite uncomfortable when your vagina is irritated from infection and/or menopause (see this chapter).

Since the speculum exam is quite uncomfortable for virgins and lesbians who have never been penetrated, it is generally reserved for those with bleeding problems.

A virgin with a bleeding problem can tolerate a speculum exam however, since the hymen is rarely intact by early adolescence due to normal straddling-type physical activity and tampon use. To demonstrate this, I often give virgins a Q-tip to slide in and out of their vaginas. The bleeding and/or spotting after your first intercourse is due to further tearing and stretching of the remnants of your hymenal ring, not an intact hymen.

You do not need a speculum exam if you have never been penetrated by a penis, tongue, finger, vibrator or dildo and do not have a bleeding problem. You may need a one-finger rectal exam however, to feel for your cervix and possibly your uterus, tubes or ovaries.

Your speculum exam can be better tolerated if you breathe deeply, lie flat without arching your back and DO NOT SQUEEZE your vaginal muscles around it. This will only make you feel it more! Remember, I have had my own speculum exams so I know what it feels like.

At this time, I would like to take this opportunity to apologize to all of you who have had pubic hair caught in a speculum. In our defense though, it is rather hard to avoid.

BIMANUAL EXAM

BIMANUAL or BM is the third part of your pelvic exam. Two fingertips are placed along either side of your cervix then gently wiggled to see if you are tender. Despite a usual warning that you are supposed to feel this, some women misinterpret any movement as pain and jump unnecessarily. Generally, we can tell who is truly tender and who is not

Next the fingertips are placed below your cervix while the other hand is placed on your lower abdomen. Gentle pressure is then applied to feel your:

1. **Uterus in the middle** to determine if it is also tender and its size. Its position is also noted as being tilted forward, straight or tilted backward, which is a normal finding in 25% of all women—myself included—and its texture is noted as being smooth or bumpy from fibroids (see this chapter).
2. **Adnexa or tube and ovary on either side of your uterus** for tenderness and any enlarged masses.
3. **Any sagging of your uterus, urethra and bladder above or rectum below.** Sometimes you have to cough with a full bladder while also standing with one foot up on a stool for us to detect this.

Since your bladder, rectum and portions of your large and small bowel are also located in your pelvis, any of them can also cause tenderness during your BM **when irritated and/or inflamed.**

It is harder to feel your uterus, tubes and ovaries if your bladder is full, tense up your abdominal wall muscles and/or have lots of abdominal wall fat, gas or stool in your bowels.

The BM does not have to be performed again when repeating the PAP if it was okay during your prior exam and PAP.

Again, you always have the option of refusing the BM exam at your own risk!

RECTOVAGINAL

RECTOVAGINAL or RV is the last part of your pelvic exam. After changing gloves, we place one finger in your vagina and another in your rectum. Then we quickly sweep them from right-to-left to check for:

1. **Bead-like nodules** that could be endometriosis (see this chapter).
2. **Hemorrhoids** in your rectum.

3. **Masses in the pouch behind your uterus** and in front of your rectum that could be an ovary, the top portion of a uterus that is titled backwards or a fibroid on a stalk.
4. **A loose muscle** that was torn after childbirth or sex.
5. **More tenderness** than the usual discomfort.
6. **Stool** amount and consistency.

Both fingers are removed and the rectal finger is checked for stool or mucus. The color is noted before smearing it onto a special card that checks for blood.

YOU DO NOT NEED A RV EXAM if you are 34 or less with a normal BM. exam, no pain nor rectal complaints.

Again, you always have the option of refusing the RVat your own risk!

REASSURING WORDS

As scary as this sounds, your first pelvic exam does not have to be a gruesome. If you relax, breathe deeply, stay still and do not tense up, your pelvic exam will probably be completed in a minute or two.

Part II

Menstrual Topics

3

Menstrual Cycle

The menstrual cycle is a topic every woman has an opinion about. A blessing for some and a curse for most; what has not been said about it. Adding my two cents to the pot, two versions are provided for you here.

The first version is simplified for those of you who do not have menstrual problems.

The second version is considerably detailed for those of you who have premenstrual symptoms, excruciatingly painful periods or an imbalance of hormones that results in difficulty getting pregnant, missed periods, abnormal bleeding, perimenopause or menopause.

SIMPLIFIED VERSION

Your menstrual cycle begins with the first day of your period, which is the first day of your FOLLICULAR PHASE as well. Typically, this lasts 14 days though it could be as short as 10 days. During this phase, a FOLLICULAR CYST or sac of fluid inside your ovary develops an immature egg FOLLICLE while also producing ESTROGEN sex hormone, which travels to your uterus to build up its inner endometrial lining for a potential pregnancy.

OVULATION or release of your follicle through its cyst wall typically occurs 15 days after the first day of your period though it could occur as early as 11 days.

This is the first day of your OVULATORY PHASE, which typically lasts 14 days with a range of 11 to 17 days. The release site heals over to form an OVULATORY CYST, which automatically dies 9 to 11 days after producing PROGESTERONE sex hormone in addition to estrogen. This further prepares your lining by slowing down its growth while ripening it for orderly bleeding later on.

MENSTRUATION occurs 24 to 28 days after the first day of your period when your lining sloughs off 2 to 3 days after its death from starvation when your nuturing sex hormone levels plummet in response to the death of your ovulatory cyst.

At the same time, your body absorbs the fluid in this cyst over the next few days while other ovary starts the cycle all over again with a new one.

You may want to skip the Detailed Version and go on to Cycle Definitions at the end.

DETAILED VERSION

Again, this version is for those of you with menstrual-related problems since the last thing you want to hear from a "Hit-and-Run" gynecologist is, "It's too complicated to explain." Well, those complicated details are the key to understanding your problem, tests that may or may not by sent by your doctor to diagnose and monitor it and any treatments that are given. To help you get through them, I have divided this version into several sections. Do not be surprised if you get lost however, since I still get lost myself!

FOLLICULAR PHASE (also called PROLIFERATIVE)

Between ages 9 and 17, the HYPOTHALAMUS **area of your brain starts to release** GONADAL RELEASING HORMONE **or** GnRH. **Your first period follows** a few weeks later.

Again, each menstrual cycle begins with the first day of your period, which is the first day of your FOLLICULAR PHASE **as well. Again, typically this lasts 14 days** though it could be as short as 10 days. During this phase, GnRH travels a short distance to the peanut-sized PITUITARY GLAND right below your hypothalamus and tells it to release FSH or FOLLICLE-STIMULATING HORMONE.

FSH travels a greater distance down to one of your ovaries where it orchestrates the development of an immature egg FOLLICLE **inside a follicular** CYST **or sac of fluid while simultaneously producing** ESTROGEN **sex hormone, which:**

1. Builds up the endometrial lining inside your uterus.
2. Makes your cervical mucus clear, thin and stretchy like egg white while also increasing mucus output from your vagina, Bartholin's and Skene's glands.
3. Makes your pituitary release LH or LUTEINIZING HORMONE while also slowing own further FSH release.

Thirteen days after the first day of your period there is a critical estrogen surge that often makes your nipples sensitive and breast tender.

Fourteen days after the first day of your period there is a similar LH surge, which is detected by ovulation kits that you buy in a drugstore.

This LH surge is followed by a third FSH surge a few hours later.

OVULATION

All three surges are necessary for OVULATION or release of your follicle through the wall of this thumbnail-sized cyst typically 15 days after the first day of your period though it could be as early as 11 days. For those of you using drugstore kits, ovulation consistently occurs 36 hours after the onset of your LH surge. The finger-like ends of your tube quickly sweep this mature follicle up.

Ovulation is a normal event that is well tolerated by 99.9% of billions of women despite the mild discomfort you may feel on the side involved. If you were born with a rare bleeding disorder however, ovulation could lead to significant blood loss and pain that generally requires emergency surgery.

Your cervical mucus has now reached its peak amount and ability to stretch in order to help sperm trying to get up inside your uterus.

Estrogen quickly falls again so your nipple and breast tenderness improve.

OVULATORY PHASE (also called SECRETORY)

This is the first day of the OVULATORY PHASE, which typically lasts 14 days with a range of 11 to 17 days. The release site heals over and accumulates even more fluid to form an even larger OVULATORY CYST. This continues to make estrogen while also producing PROGESTERONE, a new sex hormone that:

1. Slows down LH release from your pituitary while estrogen continues to slow down FSH release.
2. Makes your cervical mucus scant, white and thick enough to keep sperm from entering your uterus.
3. Further prepares your endometrial lining by slowing down its growth while ripening it for orderly bleeding later on.

PREGNANCY

Pregnancy occurs in the tube when sperm enters your follicle within 24 hours of its release. Generally, sperm generally lives for 48 to 72 hours and you are more likely to get pregnant if you have sex less than 72 hours before ovulation.

It grows over the next 5 to 7 while traveling down your tube, then IMPLANTS or buries itself into your lush prepared uterine lining. Although mild bleeding or spotting can occur at this time, it should not be mistaken for period.

Another 5 to 7 days later your implanted pregnancy begins to produce HCG or Human Chorionic Gonadotrophin, which can be detected as early as a week after ovulation on sensitive blood testing.

PREMENSTRUAL SYMPTOMS

PMS or premenstrual symptoms make most of us crazy 7 to 10 days before our periods. Numerous theories have been proposed, numerous studies done and numerous treatments tried, but there is still no one cause to explain it! It is a very confusing topic that gynecologists do not have a definitive answer for. Having experienced it myself however, I sense that many women have trouble adjusting to the see-saw effect of both sex hormones suddenly going up then suddenly coming back down again.

Specifically speaking, estrogen resembles a double-humped camel (see Figure 2.) over your cycle by surging thirteen days or so after the first day of your period, dramatically dropping a day or two later, gradually rising again from the sixteenth to twenty-second day then falling again from the twenty-third to twenty-seventh day.

Progesterone is the bigger culprit however, with a much larger single hump that begins to rise fifteen days or so after the first day of your period and reaches a gigantic peak by the twenty-first day before dramatically plunging 2 to 5 days later!

Typical premenstrual symptoms include:

1. **Weight gain from water retention, increased thirst and food cravings** due to the effect of progesterone.
2. **A resumption in nipple sensitivity and breast tenderness** due to the second estrogen rise as well as water retention from progesterone.
3. **Heaviness or a throbbing sensation in your lower abdomen,** particularly after sex, as your ovulatory cyst reaches its maximum size. Even so, it is only as big as a ping-pong and, try as you may, you cannot feel it by pressing on your lower abdomen. Ovulatory cysts rarely rupture, but when they do you can lose a lot of blood since they have an extensive network of blood vessels. Again, you may also have a lot of pain and emergency surgery may be needed.
4. **A myriad of mood changes with irritability, anxiety and depression** being the most common.
5. **Other non-specific symptoms like headache, fatigue and poor concentration.**

A PMS diagnosis requires only one of these symptoms as long as it disappears shortly after your period begins in the follicular phase.

A PMDD or PREMENSTRUAL DYSPHORIC DISORDER diagnosis however, is made when you have a preponderance of mood changes that significantly interfere with your personal and/or work relationships.

To confirm either, we encourage you to write down the dates that you experience these symptoms along with the dates of your period.

By definition, PMS/PMDD cannot be diagnosed if your periods are irregular from not ovulating. Your symptoms are considered to be PMS-like, however.

Herbal treatments have been touted, but none have been adequately studied to see if they work better than dummy pills, which typically cause 30% to improve.

Adequately studied, but not effective are progesterone, primrose oil, thyroid hormone and lithium compared to empty "dummy" pills.

Clearly effective are combined-hormone birth control pills with the same dosage of estrogen and progesterone in pills 1 to 21, Vitamin B6, Calcium and carbohydrate-rich beverages every 4 hours. Weight gain was seen with the latter, however.

SEROTONIN brain hormone boosters like Prozac, Paxil and Wellbutrin are 80% effective for PMDD as is Clomipramine, an anti-depressant, and Xanax, a Valium-related anti-anxiety a drug that is rarely used since it is frequently abused.

As a last resort, you can shut down ovarian hormone production by either removing your ovaries or having expensive monthly injections of Lupron (see the Endometriosis Chapter). Of course, both result in uncomfortable menopausal (see the Perimenopause to Menopause Chapter) symptoms that necessitate ADD-BACK menopausal hormone therapy. Unfortunately, this can bring your PMS symptoms back.

Fortunately, estrogen and related drugs like Raloxifene trigger far less PMS than progesterones like Provera or Medroxy-Progesterone Acetate (MPA) though Promethium or Oral Micronized Progesterone (OMP) and Norgestimate trigger less.

Spironolactone often helps if water retention is your only problem since this is an anti-hormone drug that also makes you pee out excess water.

Parlodel often helps if breast tenderness is your only problem since this drug lowers your PROLACTIN breast hormone (see the Anovulation Chapter).

Additionally, it makes sense to exercise, to avoid alcohol, caffeine, meal skipping and to immerse yourself in other positive lifestyle changes during this stressful time.

Personally, my favorite PMS treatment is the combined pill since it gives you a steady amount of both sex hormones without any dramatic ups-and-downs while also keeping you from making ovulatory cysts.

Figure 2. MENSTRUAL CYCLE HORMONE CHANGES

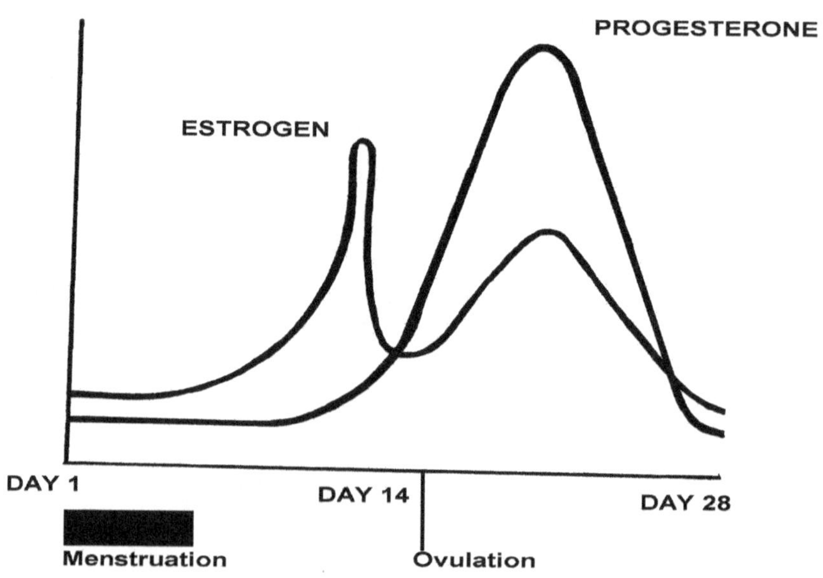

MENSTRUATION

MENSTRUATION occurs 24 to 28 days after the first day of your period when your lining sloughs off 2 to 3 days after its death from starvation when your nuturing sex hormone levels plummet in response to the death of your ovulatory cyst, which only lives 9 to 11 days.

Actually, PROSTAGLANDINS invade your lining, break it down, then causes the outer muscle layer of your uterus to contract or cramp in order to push it out. Medications like Aspirin, Naproxen/Anaprox, Ibuprofen/Motrin and its many derivatives help with cramps by decreasing your prostaglandin levels. They work better if you start them 2 to 3 days before bleeding actually starts.

At the same time, your body absorbs the fluid in your ovulatory cyst over the next few days while your brain sends down more FSH to start the cycle all over again on your other ovary.

It is impossible to have a period after you get pregnant because HCG extends the life of your ovulatory cyst. Therefore, it continues to produce sex hormones that feed your pregnancy and its lush lining. Although spotting and/or bleeding occurs often enough during pregnancy, it is due to a myriad of other causes, not a period.

Now if you thought that was hard to get through, just think about your poor body! No wonder your periods are always getting screwed up! As you can see, there are endless possibilities for things to go wrong as they often do!

CYCLE DEFINITIONS

I have provided some common definitions we use in describing the menstrual cycle to help you explain any bleeding difficulties to your medical professional.

CYCLE LENGTH is the number of days from the first day of one period to the first day of the next and ranges from 24 to 35 days.

1. Please write down the dates of any days that you bleeding, spotting or staining along with any dates you had sex and any hormones you are taking.
2. Please do not tell your gynecologist that you are having periods "twice in a month" without dates to clarify this. Eleven months have 30 or 31 days, not 28. Therefore, it is not unusual to get periods twice in a month.
3. Do not be surprised if your gynecologist is not interested in the number of days of no bleeding in-between because this is not important to us.

CYCLE DURATION is the number of days that you bleed, normally 2 to 8. This *is* important to us.

DYSMENORRHEA is an excruciatingly painful period.

INTERMENSTRUAL BLEEDING occurs on days other than your period.

MENORRHAGIA is heavy blood flow during regular periods. This is hard to measure per se, but having to change a tampon or pad every 2 hours or passing blood clots that are larger than a quarter probable qualifies.

MENOMETRORRHAGIA is heavy bleeding that is so irregular that the timing of your period is unclear.

POLYMENORRHEA are frequent periods less than 24 days apart.

OLIGOMENORRHEA are infrequent periods greater than 35 days apart.

HYPOMENORRHEA is light blood flow.

PERIMENOPAUSE is the 2 to 8-year period of ovarian decline beginning around age 46 when your periods become irregular.

MENOPAUSE is no bleeding for 6 to 12 months in a woman over 45 after your ovaries stop functioning completely.

4

Birth Control

Believe it or not, 50% of US pregnancies are unintended due to a lack of birth control! Just tune into any daytime talk show and listen to the multitudes exclaim, "It just happened." when asked how their pregnancies came about. As we all know, pregnancy does not "just happen" since there is no immaculate conception!

Among women using birth control, 33% choose hormonal methods that employ sex hormones made outside of your body. For more on sex hormones, please read the Detailed Version of the Menstrual Cycle Chapter if you jumped into the book here.

Hormonal birth control methods include:

Birth control pills, which include Combined-Hormone Pills and Mini-Pills.

Injectable agents, which include Depo-Provera shots and Lunelle shots.

Norplant upper arm skin implants.

Progestasert-IUD or INTRA-UTERINE DEVICE

For the most part, this chapter deals mostly with combined-hormone pills given the on-going bias against them and my counter-bias towards them after 22 years of use.

Although the Copper-T 380A IUD, sterilization and remaining non-hormonal methods are mentioned at the end, I apologize for turning into a "Hit-and-Run" gynecologist and glossing over the remaining methods.

COMBINED-HORMONE BIRTH CONTROL PILLS

COMBINED-HORMONE PILLS that contain estrogen and progesterone are chosen by 24%. They keep your ovaries from making eggs as well as cysts that contain them since estrogen blocks FSH and progesterone blocks LH.

Additionally, progesterone is always stronger than estrogen in any combined pill so your cervical mucus is scant and thick enough to block sperm and your uterine lining is too sparse to support a pregnancy.

The instruction book, audiotape or insert sheet that comes with your pill tells you what hormones they contain and their dosages, how to take your pills, what to do if you forget them and a lot of other information that is also mentioned in the rest of this section. Make sure you do not leave the office, clinic or ER without some type of instruction information or ask your pharmacist if you receive your pills there.

There are 8 pill-progesterones, which are listed below.

Norethindrone	Lynestrenol
Norethindrone acetate	Levonorgestrel
Norethynodrel	Desogestrel
Ethynodiol diacetate	Norgestimate

There are 2 pill-estrogens with Ethinyl Estradiol or EE being found in 49 brand-name pills and Mestranol in the remaining five.

Dosages range from 0.05 to 1.5 milligrams (mg) of progesterone and 10 to 50 micrograms (mcg) of estrogen.

Pills 1 to 21 contain hormones while pills 22 to 28 do not in 53 brand-name pills with Micrette being unique in having a half-dose of estrogen in pills 24 to 28.

There are 29 brand-name pills with hormone dose changes during pills 1 to 21.

There are really too many brand-name pills—not to mention generic—to list all of their hormone contents and dosages.

You are supposed to get a pill-period sometime during pills 22 to 28 when the lining that was previously being fed hormones during pills 1 to 21 now starves, dies and sloughs off 2 to 3 days after starting this last hormone-free week of pills.

At the same time, your pituitary detects a lack of estrogen and sends FSH down to your ovary. It then forms a tiny cyst that produces just enough estrogen to re-build your lining and keep you from having menopausal-like hot flushes. There is no increase in its size and no significant egg development over this week, however.

If you miss the first few pills however, this cyst will enlarge, produce more estrogen, and possibly release its egg. If you miss several pills in a row later on, a new cyst may form in much the same fashion. Unfortunately, taking your pill on time thereafter is no guarantee either cyst will shut down before egg release.

Well-established studies show a 0.1% FAILURE RATE when combined pills are given at the same time every day by medical personnel. This rises to 2.5% however, when you take them on your own and do not take them on time and/or miss them.

TRANSLATION: You do not get pregnant on the pill! You get pregnant by not taking it correctly!

COMBINED PILL STARTING TIMES

You can start the first pill on the FIRST DAY of your next period or same day that an abortion is performed. If you miss the first day you

can still start it on the second, third, fourth or fifth day after a period begins or an abortion.

You can also start the first pill on the FIRST SUNDAY after your next period or abortion. If this is more than 6 days since the beginning of the period or abortion, a barrier method of birth control should also be used for the first 2 weeks.

You can start the first pill 2 OR MORE WEEKS AFTER CHILD-BIRTH even if you are breast-feeding and, again, a barrier method should also be used for 2 weeks.

COMBINED PILL BENEFITS

Combined pills are so good for your period that I call them "menstrual regulation pills" and not just "birth control pills"! You will notice that your periods are more regular with less blood flow, less cramps and less PMS before because more consistent amounts of both hormones are being given and your lining growth is sparse since the progesterone is always stronger than the estrogen.

They slow down fibroid growth and lower your risk of uterine lining cancer since progesterone counteracts the harmful effects of estrogen that causes both.

Since no ovarian cysts are being made your risk of ovarian cancer is low.

You make less breast cysts since progesterone slows down their growth as well.

Your risk of uterine and tubal infections is lower since it is harder for disease-carrying semen and sperm to past through your thickened cervical mucus.

There is less acne and facial hair, particularly if you are on the latest pills containing the newest progesterones, Desogestrel and Norgestimate, since they differ from the older progesterones that strongly resemble TESTOSTERONE, the male-like sex hormone that triggers both.

If you are epileptic, you will probably have fewer seizures since progesterone lessens them.

Epileptics on Phenobarbital, Phenytoin/Dilantin, Carbazepine/ Tegretol, Oxcarbazepine/ Trileptal and Topiramate/Topamax however, may require one of the four higher-dose 50mcgEE-pills, especially if pregnancy occurred on a regular-dose 30mcg to 35mcg EE-pill. Unfortunately, these seizure medications make your liver so efficient at processing and breaking down pill-hormones that there is often too little around to keep your ovaries from making eggs and the cysts that contain them.

SIGNIFICANT COMBINED PILL RISKS

NON-FATAL BLOOD CLOTS IN A DEEP LEG VEIN or another major vein is the most significant risk of combined pills. These are fatal in 1% if a piece of the clot breaks off, gets stuck in your lungs and cuts off your oxygen supply! When you have a leg blood clot, your calf swells up and severe pain keeps you from being able to point your toes towards your head. Minor leg cramps are not necessarily a sign of leg clots.

Estrogen triggers these clots and the more estrogen you have, the more likely you are to form them. For instance, for every 100,000 women these clots will form in:

1. 48-60 PREGNANT women who have the highest levels of estrogen and this is why combined pills are begun >2 weeks after childbirth.
2. 12-20 COMBINED PILL USERS.
3. 8 OBESE non-pregnant women since fat cells takes pre-hormone substances from the bloodstream and turns them into extra estrogen.
4. 4-5 NORMAL WEIGHT non-pregnant women.

Genetics also trigger these clots since 50% of them occur in only 6% of the female population who have clotting disorders. Since most of this 6% never form clots however, there is no routine testing for these clotting disorders unless you develop them during a pregnancy or just after one or unless they run in your family.

Clots are unlikely if you have taken combined pills before or delivered a baby since you have already been exposed to comparable levels of estrogen.

A SLIGHT BLOOD PRESSURE RISE OCCURS IN 5% of combined pill users so it is generally repeated a few weeks after you start them. If this rise is significant and also persists, they are usually stopped and another birth control method is suggested. Even so, combined pills can be given to women with high blood pressure as long as it is well controlled with diet and/or medication.

THERE IS A SMALL 20% INCREASE IN EARLY BREAST CANCER before age 40 if you were on combined pills for 20 or more years. This category includes me and this increase persists for 5 years after you stop them. Even so, this translates into very few women since women under 40 make up only 4.7% of new breast cancer cases.

PRE-EXISTING GALLBLADDER PROBLEMS MAY BE AGGRAVATED during your first year on the pill use though it does not cause them per se.

MINOR COMBINED PILL SIDE EFFECTS

YOU COULD HAVE BTB OR BREAK-THROUGH BLEEDING, which is bleeding and/or spotting during pills 1 to 21.

BTB typically happens when you first start your pills do not take them on time. When you take your pill late, portions of your lining starve, die and slough off as bleeding and/or spotting.

This type of BTB is treated by simply taking your pills ON TIME during the same 2-to 3-hour time period after first performing a pregnancy test to exclude this possibility. If you are unable to do this, we suggest another method!

BTB also happens if you end up with so little lining after being on the pill for a while that it becomes fragile, unstable and prone to breaking off and bleeding at any time. Again, this is due to the effect of the stronger progesterone over the weaker estrogen.

In addition to bleeding and/or spotting during pills 1 to 21, this can also result in heavier than usual pill-period bleeding that often continues past pill 28. I have personally experienced the latter three times over my past 22 years of pill-use.

This type of BTB also requires a test for pregnancy though this is unlikely if you were taking your pills during the same 2-to 3-hour time-period.

Pills prone to this type of BTB typically have very low 10 to 20mcg doses of EE-estrogen, high-dose Norethindrone, Norethindrone acetate or Ethynodiol diacetate progesterone or a hormone dose changes during pills 1 to 21.

This type of BTB is treated with a WEEK OF EXTRA ESTROGEN, for a pack or two in order to stabilize your lining by building it back up. Typically it is begun the next time you experience BTB on your current pack of pills with the equivalent of 10mcg daily EE-estrogen or Estinyl being prescribed in the form of Premarin 1.25mg daily or Estrace 2mg daily for a pack or two.

If you are also on a pill that is prone to BTB, your next pack is then switched to one that has the usual 30mcg to 35mcg EE-estrogen dose without any high-dose progesterones or hormone dose-changes during pills 1 to 21.

The most stable pills that meet these requirements are Nordette, LoOvral, OrthoCyclen and OrthoCept, which is also known as Desogen and Marvelon. Any pill however, can result in BTB if you have been on it long enough.

Switching your pill without a week of stabilizing estrogen RARELY WORKS!

Neither does taking 2 to 4 pills a day since your lining is further destabilized **by 2 to 4 times more progesterone.**

Switching to a 50mcg EE-estrogen pill is not worth the increased risk of leg blood clots, especially since 2 of these 4 pill brands-Ovcon 50 and Ovral-have a compensatory increase in progesterone that more than matches the estrogen increase.

YOUR PILL-PERIODS COULD STOP if you end up with no lining at all as a result of a particularly strong or prolonged progesterone effect. No treatment is required since pill-periods are not a medical necessity though you should still have a pregnancy test. If you are uncomfortable with this, we can prescribe a week of extra estrogen for a pack or two while you continue your current pack, then change it to one that has 30mcg to 40mcg EE and/or no Norethindrone, Norethindrone acetate or Ethynodiol diacetate.

YOU COULD BECOME NAUSEOUS FROM THE ESTROGEN in your pill, especially when you take it early in the morning on an empty stomach. This only gives you "Morning Sickness" and I recommend taking it at bedtime to avoid this.

YOU COULD EXPERIENCE HEADACHES during the last week if the blood vessels in your brain react to the sudden hormone drop. To avoid this, you may want to switch to Micrette, which has a half-dose of estrogen in pills 24 to 28, or you may want to take your pill CONTINUOUSLY, which means starting a fresh pack every 21 days without the hormone-free break.

Sometimes they occur during pills 1 to 21 if there is a hormone dose change. To get around this, you can switch to one that has that same hormone dose in pills 1 to 21. Also, try your pill at bedtime since you are more likely to sleep through them then.

Incidentally, the effect of combined pills on migraine sufferers is unclear since 33% get better, 33% show no change and 33% get worse. If you have classic migraines with sensory auras before them, you might fall into the last category and since your risk of stroke is already increased risk of stroke whether you are on the pill or not, you may want to consider a very low-dose 10mcg to 20 mcg EE pill like Micrette with very careful monitoring or a progesterone-only birth control method instead.

YOUR SEX DRIVE MAY BE LOWER if EE-estrogen lowers your testosterone. Emotional and relationship factors are often the true cause of this, however.

THERE ARE VERY FEW WOMEN WHO CANNOT TAKE THE PILL. There are a lot of women however, who really do not want to take it and come up with every excuse in the book not to instead of just admitting this. Out of the 32 pill brands available, I am sure there is at least one that is right for you and this I say from experience. As a college freshman, I swore off the pill after my first experience with them. Five years later as a medical student, I stubbornly sat all day in the Student Health Center demanding an IUD when they offered the pill to me instead. Fortunately, they had a lot more sense than did and refused to give in to me. I was forced take the pill again and 22 years later I have never been happier.

COMBINED PILL MYTHS

Myths about combined pills needlessly keep many women from using them so lets get down to the nitty-gritty and discuss them.

You do not gain weight gain on the newer pills that contain Desogestrel or Norgestimate because these progesterones are associated with less water retention and little or no increase in appetite. You gain weight from poor food choices and a lack of exercise, but it is a lot easier to blame the pill than to admit this! I should know since I have gained weight and lost it over the past 20 years without ever stopping my pills. Discontinuing your pill for this bogus reason could result in pregnancy and this definitely makes you gain weight!

Combined pills no longer increase your risk of heart attack or stroke according to latest studies from the 1980's. By then, women with uncontrolled high blood pressure and smokers over age 35 were no longer being given them. Also, pills with 50mcg or more EE were virtually out of use. These 3 factors were associated with heart attack and stroke when the combined pills first came out in the1960's.

Combined pills no longer increase your risk of diabetes or yeast infections since the dose of estrogen is much lower these days. When combined pills first came out in the 1960's, they typically had dramatically higher 80mcg to 150mcg doses of estrogen as well as 9mg to 10mg doses of progesterone.

Combined pills have no lasting effect on your menstrual cycle after you stop them since pill-hormones are completely gone from your body within 36 hours or so. Even so, it could take a month or two for your ovaries to make enough estrogen and build up your lining for a period if they had stopped on the pill. Other future menstrual problems are not due to the pill, however. There is no need to take a "break from the pill" since you get a one-week break for every 28 days that you use it with the sole exception of Micrette. It is perfectly safe to take the pill for months, years or even decades as I have.

Combined pills are still effective when you take regular antibiotics. Special TB medications like Rifampin and Rifambutin make them less effective, however.

Combined pill can still be taken if you have varicose and/or spider leg veins since the risk of leg blood clots is the same compared to women without them.

Combined pills do not cause birth defects if you take it while pregnant.

COMBINED PILL CONTRAINDICATIONS

Generally, we do not prescribe combined pills if you:

1. **Smoke and are also 35 or older** since the combination of both increases your risk of heart attack and stroke!

2. **Have uncontrolled high blood pressure** with a similar increased risk of heart attack and stroke (though combined pills can be given if it is controlled).
3. **Have had a heart attack, stroke or a blood clot** that required blood-thinners.
4. **Have any conditions that predispose to all 3 like lupus OR sickle cell disease, which predisposes mostly to clots, OR hereditary hyperlipidemia,** which accounts for most heart attacks in women under 40!
5. **Have chronic hepatitis** with a liver that is too weak to handle pill-hormones.
6. **Have breast and/or uterine lining cancer** that are both worsened by hormones.
7. **Have undiagnosed abnormal bleeding,** which could be due to pregnancy or uterine lining cancer after further investigation.

Putting this all in perspective, I have listed your chance of dying within one year from several activities. Keep in mind, not being on combined pills puts you at significant risk for pregnancy since barrier methods, rhythm and withdrawal are so unreliable.

1. Driving kills 1 in 6,000.
2. Pregnancy kills 1 in 11,000.
3. Smoking on combined pills kills 1 in 16,000.
4. Not smoking on combined pills kills 1 in 63,000.
5. Tubal sterilization kills 1 in 67,000.
6. IUD's kill 1 in 100,000.
7. Abortion at 9 week or less kills 1 in 260,000.
8. Tampons kill 1 in 350,000.

ALTERNATIVE WAYS TO TAKE COMBINED PILLS

You can also take combined pills CONTINUOUSLY with a fresh pack every 21 days without the hormone-free week in-between. This needlessly avoids a pill-period if you are being treated with iron for severe anemia as a result heavy bleeding or suffer from excruciatingly painful periods, especially when due to endometriosis/adenomyosis (see this chapter). Since BTB is far more common when the pill is taken this way, you should consider only 2 to 3 months of continuous pill-use then break for a pill-period.

You can also use them as EMERGENCY CONTRACEPTION or "Morning-After Pills" that must be started within 72 hours of unprotected sex. This requires Ethinyl Estradiol 200mcg with Levonorgestrel 1mg with both resulting in a lining that is too sparse to support a pregnancy. This is a lot of estrogen, so half of the pills are taken as soon as you get them and the rest 12 hours later. Half get nauseous with a quarter actually vomiting so it is a good idea to ask for anti-vomiting medication since the failure rate is already high at 25%.

The Preven kit contains four 50mcg EE / 0.5mg Levonorgestrel or Ovral pills along with a urine pregnancy test dipstick.

Other combinations that can also be used include:

1. **Eight 30mg EE-pills** (white-colored LoOvral and/or Levora, orange-colored Nordette and/or Levlen, yellow-colored Trilevelen and/or Triphasil).
2. **Ten 20mcg EE-pills** (pink-colored Levlite and/or Alesse or white-colored Micrette).

PROGESTERONE-ONLY MINI-PILLS

PROGESTERONE-ONLY MINI-PILLS are chosen by <1% and are taken continuously every day without a break. They include:

1. **0.35mg Norethindrone** in Micronor, Nor-Q-D, Noriday and Norod.
2. **0.075mg Levonorgestrel** in Ovrette or Neogest.
3. **0.5mg Ethynodial Diacetate** on Femulen.

4. **0.3mg Norgestrel** in Microval, Noregeston or Microlut.
5. **0.5mg Lynestrenol** in Exluton.
6. **0.075mg Desogestrel** in CerazetteR.

They make your cervical mucus scant, but thick enough to block sperm while also making your uterine lining too sparse to support a pregnancy. Your ovaries continue to make estrogen since FSH is not blocked and ovulation occurs on occasion since LH is not completely blocked by progesterone. The FAILURE rate is 2% to 3%.

You can start them on the FIRST DAY of your next period, the same evening after an abortion, >3 days after childbirth. Regardless of when you start them, a barrier method should always be used for the first week.

They are IDEAL for women who should not use combined pills and women who complain of a low sex drive on combined pills.

They are NOT IDEAL for postpartum Hispanic women just recovering from pregnancy-related diabetes since there is a triple risk this will return or women who already have problems with ovarian cysts since even more may appear.

MANY WOMEN STOP THEM BECAUSE OF THE SIDE EFFECTS BELOW.

1. IRREGULAR BLEEDING AND/OR SPOTTING IN THE 40% who end up with an extremely sparse and subsequently unstable lining.
2. MISSED PERIODS IN THE 20% who end up with no lining. Again, this is not a bad thing since periods are not essential when you are on hormonal birth control.
3. WEIGHT GAIN as a result of water retention and increased appetite.
4. ACNE AND INCREASED FACIAL HAIR, especially when the older progesterones that strongly resemble male-like testosterone are used.

Mini-pills can also be used for EMERGENCY CONTRACEPTION within 48 hours of unprotected sex. The Plan B kit has 2 doses of Levonorgestrel 0.75mg that are taken 12 hours apart. Again, this makes your lining too sparse to support a pregnancy. Fortunately, only 3% become nauseous so the failure rate is only 15%.

DEPO-PROVERA SHOTS

INJECTABLE DEPO-PROVERA is chosen by 5% and consists of 150mg MPA or Medroxy-Progesterone Acetate, another synthetic progesterone.

Again, it thickens cervical mucus and makes your lining sparse. There is a lot more progesterone so LH and ovulation are completely blocked. Your ovaries still make estrogen since FSH is not blocked, however. The FAILURE rate is <1%.

You can get your first shot ONE TO FIVE DAYS after the onset of your next period, abortion or birth and it is repeated every 3 months or 13 weeks. It is usually injected into the muscular portion of your upper arm or buttocks.

Depo-Provera is IDEAL for certain epileptics, migraine sufferers, women who should not take combined pills or are too unreliable to take them.

BENEFICIAL EFFECTS include less fibroid growth, less blood flow during your periods or even missed periods after the second or third shot. Again, this is a good thing since monthly periods are not a medical necessity on hormonal birth control.

SIDE EFFECTS include depression in 5% and irregular bleeding in 70% that fortunately drops to 10% by the end of the first year. Unfortunately, 57% refuse the second shot. Sometimes this irregular bleeding responds to a 2-week course of Aspirin, Ibuprofen or Naprosyn if you do not have stomach ulcers or kidney disease. These medications cut down on your prostaglandins or the substances that break your lining down before it actually bleeds. They also alleviate your cramps. Although a 2-week course of stabilizing estrogen in the form of 1.25mg daily Premarin or 2mg daily Estrace can also be tried, you usually bleed a few days after you finish it.

Additionally, some women typically gain 5 pounds a year though I have had patients who exercised and watched their diets while on it and lost weight instead.

Since your ovaries end up making less estrogen there can also be some bone loss. This has been seen in some women who used Depo-Provera for 15 or more years and some who started it as teenagers. Fortunately, you make up this bone loss when you stop it and a long-term study to look at this bone loss more closely will be ready in 2003.

Depo-Provera is gone from your body 6 to 8 months after your last shot.

LUNELLE SHOTS

INJECTABLE LUNELLE—**also called** Cyclofem **or** Cyclo-Provera—**is still awaiting FDA approval. It has only 25mg MPA with 5mg Estradiol Cypionate,** another synthetic estrogen, so irregular bleeding is less of a problem.

You are also supposed to get your first shot ONE TO FIVE DAYS **after the onset of your next period, abortion or birth, but it is repeated once a month.** You can even inject yourself by using a special needle kit.

It thickens cervical mucus, makes your lining sparse, blocks FSH, LH, and ovulation. The FAILURE rate is also <1%.

NORPLANT UPPER ARM SKIN IMPLANTS

NORPLANT IMPLANTS are chosen by <1% and consist of 6 toothpick-sized plastic rods that slowly release 216mg Levonorgestrel over 5 years. The rods are surgically placed just underneath the skin of your upper arm near the armpit within the FIRST 1 to 7 DAYS after the onset of a period, abortion or birth.

It works by thickening your cervical mucus and making your lining sparse, costs $400 to $600 and has a <1% FAILURE rate. It is IDEAL for some epileptics and migraine sufferers and other women who should not take combined pills or are too unreliable.

SIDE EFFECTS include weight gain, depression, headaches, breast tenderness acne, ovarian cysts and an irregular menstrual pattern in 80% throughout the first year. A week of stabilizing estrogen in the form of 1.25mg daily Premarin or 2mg daily Estrace often improves this. Unfortunately, only 30% are still using it by the fifth year.

PROGESTASERT-IUD (Intra-Uterine Device)

The PROGESTASERT-IUD is also chosen by <1% and slowly releases 38mg of progesterone over a year through a T-shaped plastic device about 1 inch in size that is placed inside your uterus preferably during a period. It can be placed any time including within 48 hours of unprotected sex for EMERGENCY CONTRACETION, costs over $500, thickens your cervical mucus and makes your lining sparse.

The FAILURE rate is 3%, but 24% of these are tubal pregnancies that require surgical removal! Although 76% are normal uterine pregnancies, 40 to 50% miscarry or deliver prematurely if the IUD is left so it is removed as soon as possible.

You should only consider an IUD IF YOU HAVE A CHILD AND ARE IN A MUTUALLY MONOGAMOUS RELATIONSHIP. This

means you are not having sex with anyone else, he is not having sex with anyone else and you know this for a fact! If he has sex with someone else, he could pick up Gonorrhea and/or Chlamydia (see both of these chapters) and pass either one or both of them to you during sex. After they infect your cervix, uterus and tubes, the subsequent scarring that develops could keep you from getting pregnant. IUD's factor into all of this by worsening these infections as evidenced by the extremely sick women I have taken care of who had them while mistakenly believing they were in a mutually monogamous relationship!

HIV-positive women should avoid IUD's since they are less able to fight off bacterial germ organisms that normally live in the vagina and have the same potential to cause similar uterine and tubal infections.

Otherwise, it is IDEAL for certain epileptics, migraine sufferers and other women who should not use combined pills or are too unreliable.

Since 5% of IUD's fall out of your uterus on their own, there is a plastic string at the bottom that hangs down into your vagina for you to feel for after each period.

One in every 1,000 IUD placements could perforate your result in uterus or a put a hole in it from its inner cavity clear through its outer wall. Since this can also cause serious pelvic infections, surgery is usually required to find and to remove it.

ParaGard COPPER T 380A-IUD

The COPPER T 380A-IUD has copper wire wrapped around each end of a T-shaped similar-sized plastic device that works by killing sperm inside the uterus before they enter the tubes. Since sperm meets the egg in the tubes, this makes it less suitable for emergency contraception.

It is also chosen by <1%, is similar in costs and insertion technique, but is approved for 10 years of use with a one-year FAILURE rate of

only 0.3%. Although this rises to 1.6% by 7 years, only 6% of these are tubal pregnancies.

It is unsuitable if you already have a bleeding problem since heavy periods, irregular bleeding and/or spotting and resultant cramping are common side effects that lead 5% to 15% to discontinue it within the first year. Medications that lower your prostaglandin levels sometimes help, however.

STERILIZATION

FEMALE OR MALE PERMANENT STERILIZATION is chosen by 42% and has a 1% to 3% FAILURE RATE depending on how it was done. Although many states have a 30-day waiting before surgery to give you plenty of time to think about it, 7% end up changing their minds afterwards! Some of this 7% undergo a subsequent reversal, but they are usually not very successful. Ironically, many sterilized women end up on combined pills to regulate erratic periods that commonly occurrence after your mid-30's, whether you are sterilized or not.

REMAINING METHODS

The ridiculously high FAILURE RATE of 12 to 21% for male and female condoms, diaphragm, sponge, spermicide, withdrawal or rhythm should give you pause if you are relying upon any one or a combination of these methods. Since you are basically asking to get pregnant using these methods, I think it is a disservice to discuss them! They are better than nothing however, since this results in 85% pregnancy rate.

Do not get me wrong! As an adolescent, I successfully combined rhythm with condom for several months. Both were quickly abandoned however, when I broke up with my boyfriend and made up with him just as suddenly. Of course, the makeup afterwards included the requisite passionate sex and this promptly led to a pregnancy.

And therein lies the problem. Sex is just too spontaneous for them to be reliable!

PEARLS OF WISDOM FOR YOU MALE CONDOM USERS

The 12 to 21% of you who get pregnant using male condoms have the same 12 to 21% risk of getting HIV, Gonorrhea, Chlamydia or other STD's. You are even more likely to get warts or herpes after coming in contact with skin areas not covered by them.

Remember male condoms are just thin pieces of rubber that break easy and are not worth losing your life over! Choose your partners carefully and keep in mind that you can always say "NO" to sex.

If "NO" is impossible to say, carry some VAGINAL CONTRACEPTIVE FILM or VCF with you at all times for extra protection! It comes in a neat discreet package that fits anywhere, even your bra. It is also is colorless, odorless and tasteless. Just fold the thin film over once, stuff it inside your vagina and it melts immediately.

5

Amenorrhea

AMENORRHEA IS A MISSED PERIOD not due to pregnancy or menopause.

SECONDARY AMENORRHEA

SECONDARY amenorrhea is 3 missed menstrual cycles that can extend over 6 months after you have already started menstruating. This accounts for 90% of all amenorrhea and is due to a hormone problem in 82% and a physical blockage 8%.

Secondary amenorrhea requires pregnancy testing and questioning to see if you:

1. **Have been using any hormones** like combined or mini-pills, Depo-Provera or Lupron injections, Provera or Promethium tablets, Norplant or Progestasert-IUD.
2. **Recently had any surgery on your cervix or uterus** like a LEEP, cone biopsy, D+C and/or hysteroscopy?
3. **Had any signs of an autoimmune disorder** where your immune system mistakenly attacks and kills certain organs like your

ovaries in the mistaken belief that they are infected. Lupus, rheumatoid arthritis, vitiligo, myasthenia gravis, Hashimoto's thyroiditis, idiopathic thrombocytopenia purpura (ITP) and autoimmune hemolytic anemia are all examples of these.

4. **Had any cancer chemotherapy and/or radiation treatments** that may have damaged your ovaries as well?
5. **Have been using any psychiatric medications and/or illegal drugs?**

OVULATION FAILURE AND MORE HORMONES

At this point, you may want to re-review the Detailed Version of the Menstrual Cycle Chapter since it is essential to understanding amenorrhea.

ANOVULATION or not ovulating causes 28% of secondary amenorrhea. Although this is quite common when you first start to menstruate and in the years before menopause, it is also not uncommon to miss one or two periods a year. Most of the time, you go back to ovulating on your own with a return of your periods.

However, some of you will not and this results in several hormone imbalances.

1. TOO MUCH ESTROGEN WITHOUT ANY PROGESTERONE.
2. TOO LITTLE FSH in response to too much estrogen and TOO MUCH LH in response to this lack of progesterone.
3. TOO MUCH TESTOSTERONE AND ANDROSTENEDIONE male-like ANDROGEN sex hormones in response to all of this LH.
4. EVEN MORE ESTROGEN after some of this testosterone is converted into it right there in your ovary and after some of this

androstenedione is converted into it by your fat cells. More fat results in more androstenedione being converted.

5. EVEN MORE TESTOSTERONE after the rest of this androstenedione is converted into it by your skin.

The excess estrogen makes your ENDOMETRIAL uterine lining grow so much:

1. THAT IT BECOMES TOO STABLE TO BLEED IN 50%.
2. THAT IT BECOMES HYPERPLASTIC or extremely overgrown.
3. THAT IT BECOMES CANCEROUS if your hyperplastic endometrium is not treated. Since your risk of this triples if you ovulate < 4 times a year, it is important to have an office biopsy of your endometrium or EMBX if you have not had a period for a long time. The result generally takes 2 to 3 working days and is discussed in more detail in the next chapter.
4. THAT IT TURNS INTO POLYPS, ENDOMETRIOSIS AND/OR ADENOMYOSIS. See the chapters that follow for more on these.

Excess estrogen can also make your uterine muscle cells grow into FIBROIDS.

Excess testosterone makes 70% prone to acne, excess facial hair and/or balding.

Excess androstenedione and testosterone both make your ovaries:

1. UNABLE TO RELEASE AN EGG REGULARLY EACH MONTH.
2. EVENTUALLY TRIPLE IN SIZE from producing so much androgen and accumulating so many unreleased eggs trapped inside their accompanying cysts.
3. EVENTUALLY POLYCYSTIC with multiple small cysts clustered along their edges. PCOS or Poly-Cystic Ovarian Syndrome is a poor term to substitute for anovulation since polycystic ovaries are only found in 75% of women who do not ovulate regularly with up to 25% being found in women who do. For this 75%, polycystic ovaries appear after you stop ovulating, not

before. Although anovulation also results in acne, excess facial hair and balding in 70%, it is not referred to as, "AEFHBS" or "Acne, Excess Facial Hair and Balding Syndrome".

INSULIN RESISTANCE

RESISTANCE TO INSULIN HORMONE causes 50% to 60% of all infertility since it keeps you from ovulating regularly.

YOUR PANCREAS RELEASES INSULIN AFTER A MEAL TO:

1. **Supply your organs with energy by moving CARBOHYDRATES into them.** Carbohydrates include obvious sugars like fruits, soft drinks and other sweets as well as non-obvious sugars like bread, pasta, rice and starchy vegetables.
2. **Next, insulin moves any excess carbohydrate out of your organs** for storage inside your fat cells.
3. **Lastly, insulin prevents fat release** and this is allowed only when there are no more carbohydrates or interfering insulin around.

Unfortunately, 6 to 10% of you were born with a gene that makes you release more insulin than usual after a meal. Too much insulin makes you store too much of your carbohydrates as fat by moving more than just the excess out of your organs. It is as if the extra insulin refuses to leave the party without a date, whether there are enough dates to go around or not.

Over time, YOUR ORGANS RESIST THIS EXCESS INSULIN **by blocking its entrance in order to hold on to more carbohydrates.** This is particularly true for your brain and nerves since they do not have the ability to use fat as an energy-substitute.

Unfortunately, your resistant organs run out of carbohydrates 2 to 3 hours later and they are unable to use fat as an energy-substitute since there is still too much insulin around to allow fat release.

As a result of this, your muscles do not feel like moving and your brain feels light-headed, irritable and unable to concentrate on anything other CARBS, CARBS AND MORE CARBS! Of course, this incessant craving makes you consume more carbohydrates, which are quickly absorbed while triggering even more insulin release.

Enough insulin is now around to temporarily overcome your resistance and it enters your organs once more with the desperately needed carbohydrates. Even more of them are stored as even more fat and your organs become more resistant in anticipation of the next insulin onslaught.

You develop a vicious cycle with repeated carbohydrate drops 2 to 3 hours after you eat or drink. This leads to repeated carbohydrate snacking, ever higher levels of insulin, more and more fat storage, still no fat release and worsening organ resistance.

Unfortunately, insulin resistance results in:

1. **Weight gain** from this vicious carbohydrate cycle.
2. **Diabetes before age 30 in 35 to 50% with the rest developing it later on** when their pancreas finally get tired of cranking out so much insulin. This is 5 times more common in repeat anovulators with polycystic ovaries.
3. **Too much androgen and estrogen,** after the former is converted into the latter, since excess insulin has the same effect as excess LH on your ovaries.
4. **Endometrial hyperplasia and/or cancer** from the excess estrogen.
5. **Acne, excess facial hair, balding, enlarged and/or polycystic ovaries as well as an unfavorable male-like cholesterol pattern** from the excess androgen.
6. **ACANTHOSIS NIGRICANS or velvety dark pigmentation** of your neck, armpits, breast folds and groin from too much insulin and androgen. Like polycystic ovaries, this is not specific since a few normal women also have it.
7. **High blood pressure** that is generally not seen until menopause.

8. **Early heart disease in your 40's** from your heart blood vessels being clogged with extra fat being carried through your bloodstream on its way to being stored. This is worse when you become diabetic since even more fat is finally being released from fat cells now that there is so little insulin around. Of course, the unfavorable cholesterol pattern and high blood pressure also contribute to this.

Now, this may all sound terribly distressing, but do not jump out of that window just yet! There is hope for you yet.

Obviously, since carbohydrates trigger this insulin resistance you should try to limit their intake to only 2 or 3 servings and try to consume them all at one meal. Instead of a food pyramid with most of the food servings being carbohydrates at its bottom, think of a food circle with an equal calories of protein, fats and carbohydrates that should be more of the non-sweet green leafy variety that is less insulin-provoking and less of the sweet starchy vegetable and/or grain variety.

This should normalize your insulin, lessen your organs resistance to it and improve most of the other abnormalities. If you also lower your fat and total intake of calories and exercise regularly, you are bound to lose some weight as well. You do not have to lose a ton since a 5 to 10% loss is enough to correct these abnormalities.

If your insulin resistance is particularly severe, we often prescribe diabetic pills even if you are not quite diabetic since they lower your organs resistance to it.

If your cholesterol is particularly high, you may need drugs to lower it as well.

Neither set of drugs is a cure however, so lifetime diet therapy is a must!

Well, does this sound like the story of your life? All this bad news got you down, down, down? Well pick yourself up, dust yourself off and remember there are billions of women all over the Earth with this same problem. Now, go take a tea or java break, WITHOUT CARBS OF COURSE! Okay, maybe half a teaspoon of sugar.

INSULIN RESISTANCE EVALUATION

If you do not ovulate regularly and have signs of too much androgen, you need:

1. FASTING INSULIN AND SUGAR LEVELS after not eating and/or drinking for 8 hours before.
2. 2-HOUR SUGAR LEVEL after drinking 75 grams of sweet syrupy Glucola to see if insulin resistance has progressed to the point of actual diabetes.

Insulin resistance is diagnosed when the result of the fasting insulin divided into the fasting sugar is <4.5 with a normal fasting insulin level being 10-20U/ml. You would think that a 2-hour insulin would be the best indicator of insulin resistance, but unfortunately it is not. Insulin fluctuates greatly from one minute to another when it is released in response to carbohydrates, so it is a lot harder to get an accurate reading then.

Diabetes is diagnosed when your 2-hour is 200mg/dl or more OR when your fasting sugar is 126mg/dl or more. Although a normal 2-hour is 140mg/dl or less and a normal fasting sugar is 110mg/dlor less, a 2-hour between 141-199mg/dl OR fasting sugar between 111-125mg/dl are both elevated and indicative of impending diabetes.

If your insulin and sugar results are normal, you should still be tested every year since your insulin resistance may be so mild that it is impossible to detect with our current tests. As it worsens however, your results will be eventually become abnormal.

Of course, you do not have this testing if you cannot afford it since it is safe to assume that you have insulin resistance if you have signs of too much androgen and do not ovulate regularly, especially if you are also overweight.

TOTAL TESTOSTERONE and early morning 17-OHP (Hydroxy-progesterone) blood hormone testing is also indicated if you have a lot of facial hair. If it appeared rapidly over a months and total testosterone is >200ng/dL, there is a good possibility of an extremely rare androgen-producing tumor. If 17-OHP is >300ng/dL, there is a 1% to 5% possibility of a hereditary ADRENAL GLAND problem, depending on further testing. Adrenal glands are prune-sized organs on top of each kidney, which also produce androstenedione and testosterone as well as stress and fluid balance hormones.

A more sensitive FREE TESTOSTERONE test is indicated if you do not ovulate regularly without any signs of too much androgen. Unfortunately, it costs 3 times more than the insulin resistance testing your will then need if the result is >200pg/dL, so it often makes sense to skip it and proceed directly to insulin resistance testing.

Androstenedione testing is expensive and unnecessary since testosterone is the more traditional indicator of too much androgen.

Estrogen and progesterone testing is also expensive and unnecessary since both have the potential to fluctuate greatly from one day to the next, especially if sent after a chance ovulation that occasionally occurs from time to time.

LH is still normal in 20 to 40% of repeat anovulators, so expensive FSH+LH testing should be pursued only if you are being evaluated for infertility or do not bleed after a trial of progesterone then estrogen as mentioned later on in this chapter.

Pelvic sonogram is indicated only if one or both ovaries are enlarged on exam.

Save your money for the more important stuff above and below.

MORE PITUITARY HORMONES

I know, I know! You just got used to the other hormones and now I am going to add some more to the mix! It's not my fault that the body is so complicated.

Like GnRH, TRH or THYROID-RELEASING HORMONE is released by your hypothalamus prior to traveling down to the pituitary gland right below it.

TSH or THYROID-STIMULATING HORMONE is then released prior to traveling a greater distance down to the thyroid gland in the front of your neck to start thyroid hormone production.

TRH ALSO ORCHESTRATES PROLACTIN RELEASE from your pituitary. This is especially obvious if you have HYPOTHYROIDISM and do not make thyroid hormone. Your hypothalamus tries to correct this by aggressively releasing more TRH. Your pituitary aggressively releases TSH in response to this, but also prolactin.

Prolactin travels down to your breasts where it triggers GALACT-ORRHEA or nipple leakage when not associated with childbirth and milk production when it is.

To make this confusing circle complete, too much prolactin stops GnRH from being released from your hypothalamus and this, in turn, lowers your FSH+LH.

TSH+PROLACTIN TESTING

If you do not ovulate regularly, TSH and prolactin should also be checked.

If TSH is >5mU/L, you are hypothyroid. Although this accounts for only 1% of secondary amenorrhea, it is quite easy to cure with thyroid hormone.

If prolactin is >20ng/ml, you have a pituitary TUMOR or new growth. This accounts for 7.5% of secondary amenorrhea.

You will then need a relatively inexpensive pituitary x-ray, which is also indicated is galactorrhea is present regardless of your prolactin result.

If your prolactin is between 21-100ng/ml and your x-ray is normal, you have a very small slow-growing tumor that rarely causes problems. Most of the time it is simply monitored with a yearly pituitary x-ray and prolactin level while your hormones are replaced with combined-hormone pills or some other combination of estrogen and progesterone. If you want to get pregnant or have a lot of nipple discharge however, Bromocryptine/Parlodel is prescribed instead to block prolactin release.

If your prolactin is >100ng/ml and your x-ray is not normal, you have a large tumor that requires more expensive CT and/or MRI scanning and referral to a specialist.

PROGESTERONE TREATMENT

Fortunately, progesterone normalizes your FSH, LH, estrogen, androgen, endometrium and ovaries cheaply.

Promethium or Oral Micronized Progestesterone (OMP) 300mg is prescribed as a one-time bedtime dose, Provera or Medroxy-Progesterone Acetate (MPA) 10mg is prescribed for 5 nights or you are given a 200mg shot of Progesterone in oil.

BLEEDING AND/OR SPOTTING SHOULD OCCUR 2 to 7 DAYS AFTER and any amount of bleeding counts, be it a few drops or a heavy flow! Usually, you bleed a lot and have a lot of cramps because there is a lot of lining inside that has to come out.

Rarely, you bleed 14 days afterwards if ovulation is triggered as a result of your LH being blocked enough to bring your estrogen and androgen levels down.

If you do not ovulate on a regular basis, you will need it at least 4 times a year until menopause to lower your risk of endometrial cancer.

If you also have a lot of facial and body hair you will need it at least 6 months since hair has a very long growth cycle. Some of you may even need electrolysis if there has not been a significant improvement after 6 months, however.

If pregnancy is desired, we give more Provera 10mg or Promethium 200mg for 10 to 14 consecutive nights each month. Regular ovulation often resumes as your LH is blocked for 10 to 14 nights and your androgen and estrogen levels come down.

If you do not want to get pregnant, we give you combined-hormone pills, progesterone-only mini-pills or 125mg MPA Depo-Provera shots every 3 months.

Combined-hormone pills contain far more progesterone than estrogen with the latter also blocking FSH such that there is no cyst or egg formation as well. Depo-Provera blocks LH so completely that the mid-cycle ovulatory surge is no longer possible. Mini-pills do not block LH as completely, but the progesterone in them makes it hard for sperm to get past your cervix and for any subsequent pregnancy to plant roots. Fortunately, weight gain is not seen with combined-hormone pills like all of the other progesterones.

ESTROGEN TREATMENT

If you still have not bled by the second week, you will need a trial of estrogen to see if you have a different hormone imbalance consisting of too little estrogen and too little progesterone. This results in too little lining so estrogen is given to build it up.

Typically, we prescribe Premarin 1.25mg daily or Estrace 2mg daily for 21 days. To trigger actual bleeding, we then prescribe 5 more nights of MPA 10mg or OMP 200mg to start about 17 days into this 21-day course of estrogen.

If you finally bleed or spot afterwards, you should consider combined pills or some other combination of estrogen and progesterone.

FSH+LH

If you still have not bled 2 weeks after this, you will require FSH+LH testing.

IF BOTH ARE LOW, YOU HAVE ANOREXIA OR NO OBVIOUS CAUSE with each accounting for 10% of secondary amenorrhea. Both are treated with combined pills, other combinations of estrogen and progesterone and/or fertility drugs when pregnancy is desired.

IF BOTH ARE NORMAL, YOU MAY HAVE ASHERMAN'S SYNDROME, which accounts for 7% of secondary amenorrhea. This is scar tissue that forms inside your uterine cavity after too much lining has been scraped out during a D+C or DILATATION+CURRETAGE surgical procedure for life-threatening bleeding during a miscarriage or abortion. The scar tissue blocks the flow of blood out of your uterus.

A HYSTEROSCOPY telescope is placed inside your uterine cavity to see this scar tissue, which is then cut away. Afterwards, a balloon is inserted then left inside for a week to keep it from coming back. Simultaneously, a 10-day course of antibiotics is given to prevent infection along with a 2-month course of estrogen in the form of daily Premarin 2.5mg or Estrace 4mg to build your lining back up and a week of nightly MPA 10mg or OMP 200mg to start during the third and seventh week to bring back periods.

IF BOTH ARE NORMAL, YOU MAY ALSO HAVE CERVICAL STENOSIS or scar tissue in your canal after a cone biopsy or LEEP surgery. This is rare and is often treated in the office by inserting thin metal rods of increasing size inside your canal to widen it. If severe, a stiff plastic tube might be left in for a few days and/or weeks while antibiotics and hormones are taken.

IF BOTH ARE HIGH, YOU HAVE ENTERED PREMATURE MENOPAUSE. This happens to 1% percent of women before age 40 when their ovaries stop responding to FSH or LH. Again, this is treated with combined-hormone pills or some other combination of estrogen, progesterone and possibly testosterone.

Usually, an anutoimmune disorder or cancer treatment has killed your ovaries.

If you are 30 or less however, you need a SEX CHROMOSOME GENE TEST for inter-sex disorders that also kills ovarian tissue. These account for only 0.5% of secondary amenorrhea and, sensational as it sounds, these are women too!

Most are normal XX-females with subtle FSH, LH or X-chromosome problems that have been detected on a few investigational studies.

Second most common are MOSAIC females with a DOUBLE SET OF SEX CHROMOSOMES instead of one SINGLE set of either XX-female or XY-male ones.

1. **Combined XX/XO females lack one of the extra** X-chromosomes, as indicated by the O above. This is called, "Mosaic Turner's Syndrome".
2. **Combined XY/XX females have a 25% chance of developing ovarian cancer** so their ovaries should be removed!

Third are XX-females that are missing a portion of the X-chromosome.

Fourth are XXX-females with an extra X-chromosome.

Fifth are XO-females with only one X-chromosome instead of the usual two. This is called, "Pure Turner's Syndrome" and typical characteristics include:

3. Being only 48 to 58 inches tall.
4. Short webbed neck with a low hairline in back.
5. Childlike outer female genitals because there is no puberty.

There are more obscure inter-sex disorders that are beyond the scope of this book.

PRIMARY AMENORRHEA

This is another tedious section that is well-worth skipping if you or your daughter is not affected. If you are, I am sure your gynecologist will go over the possible causes and findings below in far greater detail. This section is by no means complete since it does not cover every obscure cause of primary amenorrhea.

PRIMARY amenorrhea is not having any period by age 16 or age 14 if you do not have any other signs of puberty. This accounts for 10% of all amenorrhea.

Puberty normally begins between 8 and 12 with the growth spurt first, breast development second, pubic hair appearance third and menstruation last.

Again, this requires pregnancy testing and questioning the parents about any childhood cancer treatments the daughter may have had and other family members with confused sex at birth or late puberty.

Again, blood is sent for TSH, PROLACTIN AND FSH+LH levels.

IF FSH+LH ARE LOW, A PITUITARY MRI is indicated, especially if prolactin is >20ng/ml. Again, hypothyroidism accounts for **1%** of primary amenorrhea, no obvious cause accounts for **10%** (though most have relatives with delayed puberty), anorexia accounts for **3%**, a myriad of other pituitary and hypothalamus problems account for **16%** altogether and a hereditary adrenal gland problem accounts for **1%**.

IF FSH+LH ARE HIGH, SEX CHROMOSOME GENE TESTING is **indicated to determine if your extremely premature menopause** is due to being a:

1. **XY-male with missing testes,** which accounts for 2% of primary amenorrhea.

2. **XX-female with sickle cell anemia** (since this occurs in 20% of these girls), a **different hereditary adrenal gland problem, ovaries that are resistant** to FSH+LH or **missing ovaries.** These account for **15%** altogether.
3. **Pure Turner's Syndrome, Mosaic or some other rare inter-sex disorder** with these accounting for **26%** altogether. Again, any Mosaic with a Y-chromosome should have both ovaries removed as soon as possible since 25% develop ovarian cancer and 70% develop a deep voice, increased facial and body hair from testicular tissue imbedded inside them.

IF FSH+LH ARE NORMAL, PELVIC SONOGRAM, CT AND/OR MRI may be indicated, especially if you are a virgin since your pelvic exam will be limited to looking at the outer genitals and a rectal exam to feel for a cervix and possibly a cervix.

Sometimes, LAPAROSCOPY telescope insertion through the belly button is then required see if your internal pelvic organs are present and normal in appearance.

1. **If your anatomy is normal, you are not ovulating and need insulin resistance** testing to complete this evaluation. This accounts for **7%** of primary amenorrhea.
2. **If you do not have a vagina, you have MULLERIAN AGENESIS** or failed development of your cervix, uterus and tubes. This accounts for **14%.**
3. **If you have a thicker than normal hymen that bulges when you cough, you have an IMPERFORATE HYMEN** with old menstrual blood trapped behind it. This accounts for **0.5%** is simply treated with surgery.
4. **If you have a tissue band from one side of the vagina to the other somewhere behind the hymenal ring remnant, you have a VAGINAL SEPTUM.** This accounts for **3%** and is often treated with surgery as well.

5. **If your vagina is short vagina and missing a cervix, you have TESTICULAR FEMINIZATION or are a XY-male whose genitals never responded to testosterone made by your TESTES or balls,** which are abnormally located inside your body instead of hanging in the outside SCROTUM sac. This accounts for only 1%. Your genitals did respond to testicular ANTI-MULLERIAN HORMONE however, so your uterus or tubes, cervix and the rest of your vagina never developed. **Since only 5 to 10% develop cancer and since this rarely happens before age 25, testes removal can be delayed until puberty ends.**

6

Abnormal Bleeding

I think I can say unequivocally that bleeding like a stuck pig every month is way up there in the" Top Ten Things I Hate About Being A Woman" category! Abnormal bleeding rules so many of our lives needlessly and hopefully this chapter will help you regain some control over this.

First and foremost, all bleeding is not your period or the bleeding that normally occurs 11 to 17 days after you ovulate or release an egg.

That said, abnormal bleeding is bleeding, spotting, staining and/or sludging that occurs in-between periods as well as any increase or decrease in your usual period blood flow and/or period duration. Normal or not, you should always write down any type of bleeding, spotting, staining or sludging in a calender.

Please know that maroon, brown or black blood is not abnormal per se since bright red blood normally darkens over time as it reacts to oxygen in the atmosphere. The longer it sits inside your vagina, the darker it gets.

ANOVULATORY UTERINE BLEEDING

If you jumped into the book here, you may want to review the Detailed Version of the Menstrual Cycle Chapter as well as the Ovulation Failure and More Hormones section of the Amenorrhea Chapter. Remember, shortcuts will only result in confusion.

ANOVULATION or not ovulating causes missed periods that are frequently followed by episodes of heavy and/or irregular bleeding. Although this is quite common when your periods start and when they are ending, it is also not uncommon for most women to miss one or two periods a year. Most of the time, you go back to ovulating on your own and your periods return.

However, some of you will not and end up with no progesterone, too much androgen, too much estrogen and too much of a lining that is unstable in 30% and prone to breaking off and bleeding at any time.

This results in ANOVULATORY BLEEDING AND/OR SPOTTING that typically occurs <24 or >35 days after the first day of your prior bleeding episode.

Unfortunately, this often results in anemia and the possible need for a blood transfusion if your lining worsens to the point of endometrial hyperplasia and/or cancer.

Again, you have a triple risk of cancer if you ovulate <4 times a year as well as the additional risks of weight gain, diabetes, male-like cholesterol pattern, high blood pressure and early heart disease if you are also insulin resistant. Fortunately, a low carbohydrate/low fat diet, exercise and weight loss improves insulin resistance and its additional risks as mentioned above as well as ovulation and abnormal bleeding.

ENDOMETRIAL EVALUATION AND TREATMENT

If you are 35 or older, you will need an office lining biopsy at the least to exclude endometrial cancer, which is a real concern if bleeding and/or spotting occurs after menopause. The result takes 2 to 3 days. If the opening to your uterine cavity is blocked however, an operative procedure under anesthesia is then scheduled.

Normal linings results are PROLIFERATIVE, SECRETORY OR ATROPHIC. A proliferative lining generally occurs 10 to 14 days or less from the first day of the bleeding and/or spotting episode before, a secretory lining occurs 11 to 17 days or more and an atrophic lining occurs after menopause.

Fortunately, endometrial cancer is rarely found since only 37,400 new cases were reported in the US in 1999. Your uterus, cervix, both tubes and ovaries must be surgically removed though additional chemotherapy and/or radiation therapy are sometimes needed. When detected early, the five-year survival rate is 90% with 6,400 deaths reported in the US in 1999.

Usually, endometrial hyperplasia is found. If it is ATYPICAL in anyway however, your internal sex organs should still be removed since this is one step away from cancer! If you are young and desperately want a child, you can try 30mg Provera or MPA nightly and have your biopsy repeated 3 to 4 months later. If this fails, you can then try MPA 200mg nightly, a 1000mg shot of it once a week or switch to twice weekly 500mg Megace or Megestrol Acetate. Unfortunately, the eventual failure rate is 75%.

If your hyperplasia is NOT ATYPICAL or is otherwise indicative of not ovulating or if you are <35 without need for a biopsy, progesterone in the form of combined-hormone pills are often prescribed to start that same night since they always contain far more progesterone than estrogen. Non-atypical hyperplasia aslo requires a repeat biopsy in 3 to 4 months.

If you cannot take combined-hormone pills or are trying to get pregnant, progesterone is prescribed in the form of Provera 10mg or Promethium 200mg for 10 to 14 consecutive nights, beginning that same night again. Again, ovulation is sometimes triggered as your androgen and estrogen levels come down after being blocked for 10 to 14 nights.

IF YOU ARE BLEEDING A LOT HOWEVER, combined-hormone pills are often doubled for 5 to 7 days or the dosage of Provera or Promethium is doubled for 10 to 14 nights.

Your bleeding should slow down by the third day without necessarily stopping.

Another heavy painful period should begin 2 to 4 days after you finish, however. Remember, you accumulated this lining over several months so it will take a few months to *un*-accumulate it.

Another pack of pills is started on the fifth day of this period. This time only one combined-hormone pill is taken every day for 2 or 3 more months. Your periods should now occur during pills 22 to 28 with less blood flow with each pack. If you need birth control, you can continue the combined-hormone pill. Fortunately, it is not associated with weight gain like progesterone alone.

If you took Provera or Promethium, another 10-to 14-day course is started on the first of every month or 15 to 16 nights after the first day of your period for another 2 to 3 months. Your periods should begin 2 to 3 days after you finish each course with less blood flow after each course.

Contraceptive progesterone-only mini-pills and 150mg MPA Depo-Provera shots are rarely used for anovulatory bleeding since both have the potential to cause even more irregular bleeding and/or spotting. They are also associated with weight gain.

Did you get all that? Are you thoroughly confused now? Now you see why there are "Hit-and-Run" gynecologists. Who can explain all of that in 5 minutes or less? And just think there's more below!

ESTROGEN TREATMENT

IF BLEEDING NEVER SLOWED DOWN BY THE THIRD DAY, you may have bled so much that your original overgrown is now minimal, fragile, and also unstable and prone to breaking off and bleeding at any time.

Any type of progesterone, impending menopause and Lupron shots, which shut down your ovaries, all result in the same type of lining.

This minimal lining is treated with estrogen in the form of Premarin 1.25mg daily or daily Estrace 2mg daily for 7 to 10 days to build up and stabilize it. If your bleeding is particularly heavy, you may need Premarin 1.25mg or Estrace 2mg every 4 hours for 24 hours then the usual once daily dose for the next 6 to 9 days.

You must stop all forms of progesterone while taking this estrogen though you will need to resume it afterwards to keep your lining from becoming hyperplastic. If you were not on either before, you will need 10-night course of progesterone after.

SURGERY

If you have not responded to either hormone or if the opening to your cavity is blocked, you will need a D+C or DILATATION+CURETTAGE, preferably with a HYSTEROSCOPY. First, a narrow metal CURETTE is used to quickly scrape your cervical canal. Next, it is DILATED or widened with narrow metal rods of increasing size until a HYSTEROSCOPE can be easily inserted into your cavity. Any areas of your lining that do not appear normal can be sampled and removed along with any polyps and/or fibroids, which are both discussed below. The hysteroscope is then removed and a slightly wider curette is inserted into your cavity to scrape out the rest of your uterine lining. Again, tissue results take 2 to 3 working days.

D+C alone is quicker and cheaper, but polyps and/or fibroids are often missed since your uterine lining is scraped out in a "blind" fashion.

Both are temporary fixes at best however, since your same abnormal lining, fibroids and/or polyps often return if due to an untreated hormone imbalance.

ENDOMETRIAL ABLATION delivers extreme heat or cold to your lining in order to kill it using several devices that are inserted into your cavity. It is also a temporary fix since 40 to 50% still bleed though 90% report an overall decrease. Since scar tissue forms in your cavity afterwards, it is virtually impossible to carry a pregnancy to term or sample any leftover lining if cancer is ever suspected in the future.

Of course, hysterectomy may ultimately be required to surgically remove your entire uterus if worse comes to worse.

OTHER UTERINE BLEEDING CAUSES

Most of you know about FIBROIDS, which are discussed in their own chapter.

Most of you do not know about POLYPS or tongue-like protrusions of excess lining from your uterine cavity and/or cervical canal. They are multiple in 20% of women who have them, range in size from a pimple to a thumb and are not cancerous though a few rare cancers in elderly women are initially mistaken for them.

There are 3 types of polyps with most being HYPERPLASTIC as a result of being particularly sensitive to estrogen though resistant to progesterone. The rest are FUNCTIONAL or consistent with where you are in your menstrual cycle, be it follicular or ovulatory, or any hormones you are taking. They are usually ATROPHIC however, if you are menopausal and not on replacement hormones.

Some of them are seen hanging out of your cervix and are easy to pluck out with a clamp right there in the office.

TRANSVAGINAL pelvic sonogram often finds the rest, especially when sterile salt water is squirted into your uterine cavity to make them show up better. Fluid helps sonogram sound waves travel and fortunately this distance it short since the device is placed right up against your cervix. In contrast, transabdominal pelvic sonograms often miss polyps since there is considerable distance between your uterine cavity and the device that is placed over your urine-filled bladder. The images that are obtained from either are simply shades of black, white and gray that a trained eye can interpret. They are not TV pictures, however.

Hysteroscopy is the best way to find polyps since it is a TV picture, which also lets you to distinguish fibroids from polyps, unlike sonogram, and remove both.

HEREDITARY BLEEDING DISORDERS ARE RARE with von Willebrand's Disease (vWD) being found in 1% of Whites and a lesser percentage of non-Whites. Most girls with this are not diagnosed until they start having periods with catastrophic bleeding that does not respond hormones, transfusion or D+C!

Generally, you need to see a Hematologist for special blood testing that may need to be repeated since the results are often negative the first time around. Bleeding episodes are treated with DDAVP nasal spray and combined-hormone pills to eliminate the possibility of bleeding during ovulation and to decrease period blood flow.

LIVER DISEASE ACCOUNTS FOR MOST NON-HEREDITARY BLEEDING disorders since your liver makes a lot of very important blood clotting substances.

A TANGLE OF ABNORMAL UTERINE BLOOD VESSELS can rupture on rare occasions though generally this is discovered after hysterectomy. At other times, they are picked up by an x-ray dye test of your uterine blood vessels and a radiologist then places pellets inside of the tangle in order to plug it up.

VAGINAL AND CERVICAL BLEEDING

INFECTIONS MAKE YOUR VAGINA AND/OR CERVIX FRAGILE and thusly prone to spotting or bleeding after sex. Of course, treatment easily resolves this.

MENOPAUSE MAKES YOUR VAGINA AND CERVIX ATROPHIC or small, tight, dry and similarly fragile as well. Of course, replacement hormones resolve this.

CERVICAL CANCER **also bleeds and/or spots at any time.** If you have an obvious tumor or new growth, a biopsy is performed in the office or hospital.

If you are 35 or older, we often send an ENDOCERVICAL CURETTAGE **or** ECC **scraping of your lower cervical canal along with your endometrial biopsy** if your PAP result from 6 to 12 months ago was missing canal cells, not normal or unavailable.

7

Perimenopause to Menopause

PERIMENOPAUSE is the 2-to 8-year period when your ovaries start to decline.

MENOPAUSE is no bleeding for 6 to 12 months if you are 45 or older when your ovaries no longer produce cysts, eggs or hormones. The average age of menopause is 50 with most women experiencing it between 44 and 56.

SURGICAL MENOPAUSE or female castration occurs after surgical removal of your ovaries before you have a chance to go through natural menopause.

PREMATURE MENOPAUSE occurs at age 40 or less in only 1% of all women. Typically, this happens if are seriously ill or have undergone prior cancer treatment.

Premature menopause before age 30 is almost unheard of since it generally occurs in women who were being born with a sex chromosome genetic disorder.

OVARIAN LIFE SPAN

Again, you may want to go back the Detailed Version of the Menstrual Cycle.

Your ovaries are packed with hormone-producing egg follicles that naturally die off, so you only have about 300,000 by your first period as opposed to 2 million at birth and 6 to 7 million when you are only 5 months old inside your mother's womb.

By the time you are in your late 30's, you only have about 25,000 left since you destroy even more follicles with each menstrual cycle.

These remaining follicles are naturally resistant to FSH, having held out for decades, so your pituitary has to send down more and more FSH to get them to respond. Unfortunately when they do respond, they do so with vengeance by making more and more estrogen, but no progesterone since you also end up ovulating less and less. All of this FSH makes you destroy even more follicles.

ESTROGEN EXCESS

All this estrogen makes your uterine lining grow too much. Eventually it becomes unstable and prone to breaking off and bleeding any time.

It can even develop into far more serious endometrial hyperplasia or lining overgrowth that is particularly exuberant and capable of progressing to cancer!

Polyps and fibroids often grow as well from all of this estrogen, though the latter generally shrink after menopause when it drops.

ESTROGEN DEFICIENCY

Estrogen levels falls dramatically less that a year before actual menopause when the few follicles that are left refuse to respond to any more FSH.

Your sex organs become ATROPHIC or thin, dry and small from shrinkage. Your vagina cracks, tears and becomes prone to infection so sex is often painful with bleeding and/or spotting afterwards. Your urethra becomes unstable so you urinate a lot. Your uterine lining hardly grows so it becomes fragile, unstable and prone to breaking off and bleeding and/or spotting at any time. Eventually, it no longer grows and your periods cease. Your ovaries become as small as an almond and no longer make cysts.

You often get HOT FLUSHES or brief periods of intense body heat and perspiration that start at the top of your head prior to traveling down to your neck and chest. They last seconds to minutes, 1 to 5 years, can be rare or as frequent as every 10 to 30 minutes and tend come at night, during stress and after actual menopause. Their true cause is not known, though is known that LH surges at the same time.

You often get INSOMNIA AND DAYTIME FATIGUE from not sleeping at night when your hot flushes are typically more frequent.

You LOSE YOUR ABILITY TO CONCENTRATE since estrogen revitalizes certain areas of your brain and lessens your chances of becoming demented from Alzheimer's. It will not improve pre-existing Alzheimer's, however.

You LOSE YOUR PROTECTION AGAINST COLON CANCER, the third leading cause of cancer deaths. Estrogen users have a 35% decreased risk of this.

You LOSE BONE AND DEVELOP OSTEOPOROSIS with resultant hip, spine and wrist fractures. This affects 8 million American women and results in 1,500,000 yearly fractures with women out-numbering men 4 to 1! At age 50, half of all White women and 10% of all Black women have fractures. Asian women, thin women, smokers, women with an overactive thyroid or women on steroids are also prone to fractures. Of the 300,000 Americans who fracture a hip each year, 24% die within a year and another 24% enter a nursing home.

Your bones should be monitored on a regular basis since it takes years to develop fractures despite suffering the most bone loss 5 to 7 years after menopause. Although it is simple and cheap to measure your wrist and heel bone thickness, neither is a true representation of your spine and hips. A total body CT scan also measures your spine, but costs a lot more. DEXA or DUAL ENERGY X-RAY ABSORPTIOMETRY measures everything, your hips included, using far less radiation than all of the above.

Keeping your bones strong requires hormones, 500mg Calcium daily and weight bearing exercise like weight lifting, aerobics, jogging or stair-master. Tums, Oscal or Citocal at each meal provides the most Calcium. Massive doses of it alone are not effective without hormones to improve its absorption from your stomach and intestines.

You LOSE YOUR PROTECTION AGAINST HEART DISEASE, the number one cause of death for more than 500,000 American women each year. This is greater than the next 16 causes of death combined including breast cancer, the second most common with 43,300 American deaths in 1999. Putting this bluntly, heart disease kills 1 in 2 while breast cancer kills only 1 in 27!

Estrogen is so protective that our heart attacks occur > 20 years or so after men with only 29,000 of these deaths occurring in women between 45 and 64 and another 6,300 in women 44 or younger.

Estrogen protects by improving blood flow thru your heart vessels several ways. It makes your heart vessels wider by relaxing the muscles that are inside of their walls. It also keeps these vessels clear by raising your HDL, the "good" cholesterol that does not stick to their walls, while lowering your LDL, the "bad" cholesterol that does. It lowers other glue-like substances that stick to your vessels as well.

Estrogen may not protect you as well if you already have heart disease as 1 in 5 women do. Therefore, you still need to eat sensibly, exercise regularly, watch your weight, avoid tobacco and aggressively treat any diabetes, high blood pressure and/or high cholesterol.

ANDROGEN EFFECTS

ACNE, FACIAL HAIR, BALDNESS AND SEX DRIVE MAY INCREASE **if your ovary ends up making more than its usual 25 % contribution of testosterone** in response to the LH rise that occurs when you stop making progesterone.

YOU ARE MORE LIKELY TO HAVE A LOW SEX DRIVE HOWEVER, **since your overall testosterone is usually low when 50% of it is lost after your ovaries stop making androstenedione as well.** Some of this used to be turned into testosterone by your skin and the extra testosterone from your ovaries is generally not enough to compensate for this sizeable loss.

Fortunately, androstenedione is still being made by your ADRENAL GLANDS or prune-sized organs on top of each kidney that produce the remaining 25% of your testosterone along with mineralocorticoid hormones that maintain your fluid balance and glucocorticoid hormones like CORTISOL and ADRENALINE that manage stress.

PROFOUND FATIGUE SOMETIMES OCCURS **if your adrenals have been too sick to make their 90% contribution of** DIHYDROEPIANDROSTERONE **or DHEA, which gives you energy, vitality and helps you sleep.** Although your ovaries make the other only 10%, this is enough to compensate for sick adrenals unable to do so. When your ovaries stop making it after menopause however, you end up with none.

ESTROGEN PRODUCTION AFTER MENOPAUSE

Fortunately, fat turns the rest of your androstenedione into estrogen and the more fat you have, the more estrogen you make.

Thusly, thin women have menopause earlier from more estrogen deficiency with more atrophy, hot flashes, memory loss and osteoporosis.

Conversely, heavy women have menopause later from an excess of estrogen with more endometrial hyperplasia and/or cancer, fibroids and polyps as well as more facial hair, acne and hair loss from an excess of testosterone as well.

Sometimes a heavy woman over 50 incorrectly assumes that menopause is behind a lapse in her periods when it is actually due to an excess of estrogen, which led to excessive growth of a lining that was so stable that it failed to bleed.

To check for this, we often give Provera/MPA 10mg daily for 14 days to see if they have enough lining to bleed and/or spot afterwards. If so, a portion of their lining is biopsied to exclude endometrial hyperlasia and/or cancer.

DIAGNOSIS

You are perimenopausal when your periods are irregular from estrogen excess or estrogen deficiency. There is no need to waste your money on FSH+LH, estrogen and progesterone blood tests since they are all unreliable at this time.

You are officially menopausal if you have not had any bleeding and/or spotting for 6 to 12 months and *ALSO HAVE A FSH >20 AND LH>30*. By this time, your few remaining follicles are totally resistant to sky-high levels of FSH and ovulation is now impossible. Your ovaries are no longer capable of making any progesterone and your LH rises permanently.

Some medical professionals will only check FSH, but this is often misleading. A high FSH alone is no guarantee that you still won't ovulate on occasion and get pregnant as evidenced by the 57 year-old grand-mother who recently gave birth to triplets without fertility drugs!

TREATMENT

HRT or HORMONE REPLACEMENT THERAPY treats peri-menopause as well as menopause and is widely recommended even if there are no symptoms. This is due to the fact that there are far more deaths from heart disease and hip fractures than breast cancer and that all three can exist for years without any obvious symptoms.

HRT is only taken by 20% women eligible for it however, since there are no 20-or 30-year studies to verify that it actually prolongs life. Fortunately, a 15-year American study following 27,000 women on HRT and 68,000 not on it began in 1993 to look at this. It will not be ready until 2008 along with a similar British study in 2011.

HRT can be taken several ways. You can swallow oral or mouth tablets, insert other tablets, cream or a ring inside your vagina, apply other creams and patches to your skin or receive intravenous estrogen in certain emergencies. The best way to treat urinary and vaginal atrophy is through your vagina and you start to see improvement within the first 2 to 4 weeks though it often takes 6 to 12 months to truly return to normal. The vaginal estrogen ring is well suited for this since it lasts 3 months. Vaginal estrogen creams however, need to be inserted every 1 to 3 days and should never be used to lubricate your vagina because this increases the dose. You also apply skin creams every 1 to 3 days and most of the patches last 3 to 4 days though one lasts an entire week.

HRT comes in a variety of dosages to accommodate your varying needs. Typically you need a high dose if you underwent surgical or premature menopause in your 20's or 30's since you are used to higher hormone levels. In early perimenopause, you generally need low doses since your ovaries are still making hormones. As this progresses towards menopause however, you often need an increase in dose as your ovaries make less and less hormone. You may even need a further increase years or decades after menopause if you have osteoporosis. In general though, we try to give you the lowest dose that will resolve symptoms, preserve bone and improve cholesterol.

HRT includes natural, plant-based and synthetic hormones. Unfortunately, these 3 categories generate a lot of confusion. For example, Premarin is entirely natural since it is obtained from the urine of pregnant horses. Only half of it is identical to our hormones, however. Although plant-based hormones are also natural and somewhat familiar to us since we have been eating them for millennia, they are not identical to our hormones and have to undergo additional man-made changes to make them so. Synthetic hormones are plant-based, but no longer identical to ours after undergoing even more man-made changes to make them stronger and/or last longer.

HRT is manufactured by formulating pharmacies as well as private companies. There are over 1,500 formulating pharmacies in the US that generally produce plant-based hormones and most will mail them to you in accordance with your doctor's prescription. Of course, there are several companies that produce brand name and generic versions of natural, plant-based and synthetic hormones.

ESTROGEN REPLACEMENT THERAPY

ESTROGEN REPLACEMENT THERAPY or ERT is very effective since it lowers your risk of spinal fractures by 80%, arm and hip fractures

by 50 to 60% and heart disease by 50% to 70%. There are over 32 ERT products to choose from and more are on the way including a gel—Oestrogel-now being used in France.

Plant-based E1 or ESTRONE is the estrogen that your fat makes from androstenedione. It is of intermediate strength and is prepared by both formulating pharmacies and a few companies. Ogen and Orthoest are both brand-name versions of Estropipate, which comes in 0.625mg, 1.25mg and 2.5mg oral tablets with 1.25mg being equivalent to 0.625mg Premarin. Estratab and Menest are both brand-name versions of Esterified Estrogens, which comes in 0.3mg, 0.625mg, 1.25mg and 2.5mg oral tablets with 0.625mg being equivalent to 0.625mg Premarin.

Plant-based E2 or MICRONIZED ESTRADIOL is the estrogen made by your ovaries so it is the strongest. It accounts for 76% of estrogen prescriptions worldwide and comes in several forms. Brand-name Estrace oral tablets and vaginal cream both come in doses of 0.5mg, 1mg and 2mg, Vagifem is a 25mcg vaginal tablet and Estring is a 90-day vaginal ring. Estrace is equivalent to 0.625mg Premarin. Micronized estradiol is also made by formulating pharmacies under various other names.

E2 also comes in skin patches that often better for hot flushes than tablets since they are quickly turned into weaker E1 by your digestive system. These include weekly Climara and Estraderm and twice weekly Alora, Esclim, Estraderm, Vivelle and Vivelle-Dot. A 0.05mg/day patch or 1mg dose are both equivalent to 0.625mg Premarin.

Plant-based E3 or ESTRIOL is the estrogen that various tissues make after E1 and E2 are used up. It is the weakest so your bone and heart are not protected though your uterine lining and breasts are not stimulated to grow. Because of this, E3 has been cautiously given to a few women with advanced breast and/or endometrial cancer that has spread to other areas. It is manufactured only by formulating pharmacies.

Plant-based BI-EST has 1mg E3/0.25mg E2 and TRI-EST has 1mg E3/0.125mg 2/0.125mg E1. Both are made only by formulary pharmacies.

Again, natural CEE or CONJUGATED EQUINE ESTROGEN is brand-named Premarin in both oral tablet and vaginal cream forms. It was the first hormone to be mass-produced in 1939 using urine from pregnant horses since it was too difficult to obtain a consistent urine supply from pregnant women. Not surprisingly, it accounts for 90% of estrogen prescriptions in the US though only10% worldwide. It is also the most popular US prescription drug and has been used in >90% of menopausal studies.

CEE contains 10 different estrogens with 52.8% of it being 2 types of E1 and another 5.4% being 2 types of E2. The other 6 are not identical to ours, but some of them are still active in our bodies. Again, the standard dose is 0.625mg, though 0.3mg, 0.9mg, 1.25mg and 2.5mg doses are also available. Though bone protection is seen with all of these, the higher doses provide the most protection.

Plant-based CONJUGATED ESTROGEN is brand-named Cenestin and comes in 0.625mg, 0.9mg and 1.25mg oral tablets with 0.625mg being equivalent to 0.625mg Premarin. It contains only 9 of its estrogens though both E1's and E2's are included.

Synthetic EE or ETHINYL ESTRADIOL is the strongest estrogen of all and is brand-named Estinyl. It comes in 2mcg and 5mcg oral tablets as opposed to the 10mcg to 50mcg dosages that are used in the pill and 5mcg is equivalent to 0.625mg Premarin.

Synthetic DIENESTROL is available only as Ortho Dienestrol vaginal cream.

YOU ARE AN ERT CANDIDATE ERT if you are menopausal without your uterus or perimenopausal with hot flushes, especially if the occur during the hormone-free last week of combined-hormone pills.

ERT CAN GIVE YOU BREAST TENDERNESS AND/OR HEADACHE though this often improves when your dose is lowered or when a vaginal cream is used instead.

ERT INCREASES YOUR RISK OF ENDOMETRIAL CANCER 2 to 10 times consistently in over 40 studies worldwide! In the US in 1999, there were **37,400 new cases and 6,400 deaths due to this. Generally, we do not prescribe ERT alone if you still have your uterus, but no periods.** This applies to all forms of estrogen, be it rings, creams, patches or tablets Even so, ERT can be given safely without fear of cancer recurrence if you have Stage I+II disease confined to your uterus and cervix.

ERT PROBABLY INCREASES BREAST CANCER SLIGHTLY. I wrote "probably" because there are over 50 studies worldwide with conflicting results. It is hard to compare one study to another since they involved different numbers of women who took different types and doses of estrogens for different periods of time.

The largest and longest study that followed 69,000 nurses between 1972 and 1992, showed a 36% increase in the breast cancer risk for current users and a 46% increase for 5 to 10 years of use. A large combined analysis of 51 studies from 21 countries accounting for 52,000 women with breast cancer and 108,000 without revealed that >5 years of ERT increases your risk of breast cancer 35%. This increase translates to 1.3 to 2 opposed to the usual 1 out of 500 women at age 50 who get breast cancer. Again, the American and British studies in the works should shed more light on this.

Of course, this probable increased risk is of great concern to the 173,700 American women who were diagnosed with breast cancer in 1999 and the 43,300 who died of it then as well. Even so, ERT is cautiously being given to some breast cancer patients with severe menopausal symptoms. Please forgive me if I sound dispassionate, but my mother died of breast cancer and I assure you I am not.

ERT INCREASES YOUR RISK OF NON-FATAL LEG BLOOD CLOTS during the first year just like combined pills. Fortunately, this only occurs in 2 to 3 women out of 10,000 as opposed to 1 out of 10,000 not on ERT.

ERT WORSENS GALLSTONES during the first year just like combined pills.

ERT WORSENS HEREDITARY HYPERLIPIDEMIA, a frequent cause of heart attack before 40 just like combined pills.

ESTROGEN-PROGESTERONE REPLACEMENT THERAPY

ESTROGEN-PROGESTERONE REPLACEMENT THERAPY or EPRT **protects you against endometrial cancer, but bleeding is inevitable!** Progesterone reverses the lining growth in response to estrogen and your uterus does not care how old you are since it will react to man-made hormones just like it reacted to the hormones that your ovaries used to make by bleeding.

EPRT PROTECTS YOUR BONES BETTER THAN ERT since progesterone has its own ability to preserve bone.

PROGESTERONE ALSO HELPS WITH HOT FLASHES AND INSOMNIA since it tends to make you sleepy. Thusly, bedtime is the best time to take it.

PROGESTERONE IS COMBINED WITH ESTROGEN SEVERAL WAYS.

Plant-based 2% PROGESTERONE CREAM in a strength of 400mg per ounce results in a dose of 25mg to 30mg in ¼ teaspoon or twice that in ½ teaspoon when rubbed into your inner thighs, hips or lower abdomen at bedtime for 10 to 14 nights in a row or twice a day for 10 to 14 days in a row each month. Either dose protects your uterus from 0.625mg Premarin if Angel 1 Care, Bio Balance, Eden Cream, Equilibrium, Estro-All, Femarone-17, Fem-Gest, Happy PMS, NatraGest, Ostraderm, PhytoGest, Pro-Alo, ProBalance, Pro-G, Pro-Gest, PROGEST-1 Complex, Progonol, Pro-Oste-All, Renewed Balance and Serenity are used. The other brands often contain no hormone.

Plant-based ORAL MICRONIZED PROGESTERONE (OMP) is brand-named Promethium with the vaginal gel form being brand-named Crinone. Promethium comes in 200mg and 100mg oral capsules while Crinone comes in an 8%-90mg dose and 4%-45mg dose. To protect your uterus from 0.625mg Premarin, you need to take 100mg for 14 nights in a row or insert an 8%-90mg dose twice a day for 14 days each month.

Synthetic MPA or MEDROXY-PROGESTERONE ACETATE is brand-named Provera, Cycrin and Amen, comes in 2.5mg, 5mg and 10mg oral tablets with 5mg being equivalent to 100mg OMP and 5mg for 14 nights in a row or 2.5mg each and every night is needed to protect your uterus from 0.625mg Premarin.

Synthetic NORETHINDRONE, NORETHINDRONE ACETATE AND NORGESTIMATE are all potent pill-progesterones. Norethindrone 0.7mg and Norethindrone 1mg acetate are both equivalent to MPA 5mg.

In contrast to the other progesterones, MPA causes a lot more breast tenderness, bloating, headache and depression while also lowering the beneficial rise in "good" HDL-cholesterol that occurs in response to estrogen. Despite the latter, your cholesterol profile is still beneficial overall when MPA is a part of your EPRT regimen.

YOU ARE A CANDIDATE FOR EPRT IN THE FORM OF THE PILL if you are a perimenopausal non-smoker without high blood pressure. It provides excellent bleeding control as well as contraception with the Micrette brand being particularly good for hot flashes due to a half-dose of estrogen in pills 24 to 28.

YOU ARE A CANDIDATE FOR OTHER FORMS OF EPRT if you are menopausal with a uterus, your periods stopped while you were on ERT, you had endometriosis left inside after surgery to remove your reproductive organs or are still on combined-hormone pills past age 52 with a FSH >20 while on pill 27 or 28 at the end of the hormone-free last week. Endometriosis is uterine lining that is abnormally planted throughout your pelvic and abdominal cavities with the same potential to become cancerous on ERT as the lining inside your uterus. Also, combined pills are associated with serious complications after age 52 so we should try to switch down to menopausal hormones that are 4 to 7 times less potent at that time. Again, ERT is safe after surgery for limited Stage I and II endometrial cancer, but the addition of progesterone probably provides even more protection against cancer recurrence.

SEQUENTIAL EPRT is estrogen every day with only 14 nights of progesterone each month. Generally, we prescribe PremPhase with 0.625mg CEE daily and 5mg MPA for 14 consecutive nights each month. Sometimes we substitute 200mg OMP or 0.7mg Norethindrone for 5mg MPA and 1mg E2, 0.625mg Esterified Estrogen or 1.25mg Estropipate for 0.625mg CEE.

CONTINUOUS EPRT is estrogen every day with progesterone every day. PremPro 0.625/2.5mg contains 28 days of 0.625mg CEE and 28 nights of 2.5mg MPA with PremPro 0.625/5mg having 5mg MPA instead. Sometimes we substitute 0.35mg Norethindrone for 2.5mg MPA and 1mg E2, 0.625mg Esterified estrogen or 1.25mg Estropipate for 0.625mg CEE. Although 100mg OMP is equivalent to 5mg MPA, its capsule cannot be halved into the 50mg dose that is equivalent to 2.5mg MPA.

Synthetic Activella has 1mg E2 and 0.5mg Norethindrone acetate and FemHRT 1/5 has 5mcg EE and 1mg Norethindrone acetate. Both 1mg E2 and 5mcg EE are equivalent to 0.625mg CEE, 0.5mg Norethindrone acetate is equivalent to 2.5mg MPA though 1mg is equivalent to 5mg MPA. More of these pills are in the works as well.

You can also apply twice weekly Combipatch 0.05/0.14mg that has 0.0 5mg/day E2 and 0.14mg/day Norethindrone or Combipatch 0.05/0.25mg that has 0.25mg/day.

PULSED EPRT is estrogen every day, but progesterone for only 3 days straight then 3 days off, etc. Synthetic Ortho-Prefest has 1mg E2 in each pill and an additional 0.09mg Norgestimate in pills 4 to 6, 10 to 12, 16 to 18, 22 to 24 and 28 to 30.

AGAIN, EPRT MAKES YOU BLEED and there is not a whole lot we can do about it except try another regimen. Generally, sequential HRT has an 80 to 90% chance of bleeding that begins 2 to 3 days after the progesterone is finished. Continuous HRT has a 40 to 60% chance of irregular bleeding and/or spotting at any time though this fortunately drops to 10 to 20% by the end of the first year. Pulsed HRT has only a 10 to 20% chance of irregular bleeding and/or spotting on any given day.

HRT IRREGULAR BLEEDING IS INVESTIGATED SEVERAL WAYS.

If you or your gynecologist is anxious, if you are still bleeding beyond a year on a continuous regimen, if you bleed before your progesterone is finished on a sequential one, a VAGINAL PELVIC SONOGRAM is often done to look for polyps, fibroids and a uterine lining >4 millimeters thick. If so, an office ENDOMETRIAL BIOPSY is then performed. HYSTEROSCOPY or telescope insertion into your uterine cavity is another option, which often picks up polyps and/or fibroids that were missed on your sonogram.

Personally, I think it is unrealistic to expect your uterus not to bleed when that is all that your uterus knows how to do! You frequently end up with the same irregular bleeding and/or spotting when the birth control pill is taken in a similar continuous fashion with a fresh pack every 21 days instead of every 28 days when trying to avoid pill-periods. Being an avid 22-year combined-hormone pill user, I can't wait for a better menopausal pill to come out with perhaps 1mg E2 or 5mcg EE in pills 1 to 28, but only 0.5mg Norethindrone acetate instead of 1mg, 0.35mg Norethindrone or a comparable dose of another synthetic progesterone in pills 1 to 21. This should hopefully result in a predictable, but brief and light pill-period sometime during pills 22 to 28.

EPRT PROBABLY INCREASES BREAST CANCER AS WELL since the previously mentioned study showed a 46 % increase. This was quite a surprise since it was previously assumed that progesterone protects breast from estrogen like it does the uterine lining. Again, the pending studies should settle this issue.

PREMPRO MIGHT INCREASE YOUR HEART ATTACK RISK SLIGHTLY during the first 4 months if you already have heart disease. Fortunately, it finally lowers this risk by the second year through an increase in your "good" HDL and a decrease in your "bad" LDL. Since the reasons for the initial increase are unclear however, HRT should be given cautiously if you already have heart disease.

PROGESTERONE REPLACEMENT THERAPY

PPROGESTERONE can be given if estrogen cannot since it also improves hot flushes and preserves bone when Calcium is doubled to 1,000mg. MPA 10mg to 20mg is typically used as well as the other progesterones.

Cholesterol should be checked and your vaginal dryness may worsen, however.

DHEA REPLACEMENT THERAPY

DHEA REPLACEMENT THERAPY **can be given for the profound fatigue** associated with low levels and is available at most health-food stores.

It comes as a cream, tablet or tincture with 5 to 10mg being given twice a day though higher 25mg twice daily doses may be required on occasion.

Your sex drive may improve since some of it is turned into testosterone. Again, cholesterol should be checked since both androgens predispose to a male-like pattern.

After 3 months, your DHEA should be checked. If normal, your dose should be gradually lowered to give adrenals a chance to gradually resume their function instead of suddenly stopping it.

TESTOSTERONE REPLACEMENT THERAPY

TESTOSTERONE is the best way to improve your sex drive and/or re-vitalize atrophic outer genital skin, which does not respond well to estrogen. It also helps with vaginal atrophy if you are not able to take estrogen.

Since testosterone also frees up estrogen that is trapped and hidden away from the organs that need it, bone is further protected. It also improves hot flushes that resumed after initially responding to ERT.

Plant-based TESTOSTERONE is made only by formulating pharmacies. You can take a 0.5mg or 1mg capsules twice a day or apply 1 to 2 mg of a 0.5%, 1% or 2% cream to your skin every other night or insert it inside your vagina every other night.

AndroGel testosterone gel however, is supposed to be released Summer 2000.

Synthetic MT or METHYL TESTOSTERONE 1.25 or 2.5mg taken every other day avoids facial hair, acne, hair loss and low voice associated with the 5mg daily dose.

Synthetic MT has also been combined with Esterified Estrogens under the brand name Estratest-HS and Estratest. Estratest-HS contains 1.25mg MT and 0.625mg Esterified Estrogen while Estratest contains double doses of both.

Of course, progesterone will also be needed to protect your uterus if you are menopausal or have leftover endometriosis and cholesterol needs to be monitored.

OTHER TREATMENTS

TIBOLONE or Livial 1.25mg daily or 2.5mg daily is a new hormone pending FDA approval that is quickly broken down into estrogen, progesterone and androgen. It preserves bone while improving hot flushes, vaginal dryness and low sex drive. Bleeding can be troublesome on 1.25mg, though only 10 to 20% bleed on 2.5mg and your cholesterol should be monitored since there are no long-term studies.

RALOXIFENE or Evista 60mg daily is a new hormone with several estrogen-like features. It is an alternative osteoporosis treatment that preserves bones and reduces spinal fractures 44% though hot flashes and leg cramps can be a problem. Short-term studies suggest a good cholesterol effect and a 5-year study to determine its effects on heart disease began in 1998. Fortunately, it does not make you prone to uterine lining overgrowth and cancer like its older sister, Tamoxifen, which is used to treat breast cancer as well as to prevent it in high-risk women.

BIPHOPHONATES preserves bone and reduces fractures. DIDRONEL or Etidronate 400mg daily is taken for 2 weeks cycles with a 3-month pause for Calcium therapy before resuming it again. It is better tolerated than RISEDRONATE or Actonal 5mg daily and FOSAMAX or Alendronate 10mg daily since both are associated with ESOPHAGUS or food-pipe injuries.

CLONIDINE or Catapres-TTS 100mcg weekly skin patches helps hot flushes.

HERBAL BLACK COHOSH improves hot flushes and vaginal dryness by lowering your LH. It is also known as Cimicifuga racemosa or Remifemin and you have to take two 40mg tablets twice a day at least for 2 to 4 weeks to see an effect.

HERBAL VITEX—also known as Chasteberry—actually lowers your sex drive and has a progesterone-like effect that helps with estrogen-excess bleeding.

SOY, YAM and PEANUT products are also available, but they do not have enough phyto-estrogen to protect your bone and improve your cholesterol.

SEX HORMONE TESTING

Some of you may still want sex hormone testing if you are unsure about starting HRT or to pinpoint what type of HRT is best for you.

Like FSH+LH, it is more accurate after menopause when your hormones are no longer fluctuating.

Given its expense however, it is perfectly acceptable to start HRT without it.

A full hormone profile includes E1, E2 and E3 estrogen measurements as well as testing for progesterone, testosterone and, perhaps, DHEA and cortisol.

BLOOD AND SALIVA testing are both available, though saliva is cheapest. Blood testing is widely available, but only a few labs analyze saliva. These few labs utilize the mail to send out collection kits that are then returned with your saliva.

Saliva testing has the advantage of measuring only active hormone that is freely available to your the organs as opposed to inactive hormone that is hidden away from them. Depending on the particular test that is used, your blood results may be misleading when the measurement includes inactive as well as active hormone.

Phew, the worst is now over! I promise you, the remaining chapters are not as bad.

8

Endometriosis and Adenomyosis

ENDOMETRIOSIS is lining that is growing outside of your uterine cavity after being deposited elsewhere inside your pelvic and abdominal cavities.

ADENOMYOSIS is lining that is growing down into the underlying muscular layer of your uterus.

CAUSES

Uterine lining is deposited in your pelvic and abdominal cavities several ways.

Menstrual blood has been seen flowing out of fallopian tubes during surgery.

Endometriosis develops in women who lack certain protective factors since most of these same women with blood flowing out of their tubes never come down with it.

Lining leftover after sex organ development can be scattered throughout your pelvis and abdomen. This is borne out by men who got endometriosis after receiving high-dose estrogen therapy for prostate cancer that awakened leftover lining, which was supposed to disappear while they were still in their mother's womb.

Lining also travels through your blood vessels to distant sites and the best example of this are women whose lungs collapse during their periods from endometriosis. And you thought you had it bad!

COMPLICATIONS

The lining that is deposited in your pelvic and abdominal cavities reacts to hormones just like the lining that is normally inside your uterus with estrogen building it up and progesterone ripening and slowing down this growth. When both hormone levels drop at the end of your menstrual cycle, this lining also starves, dies and is sloughed off as a period.

This period blood however, is extremely irritating to your pelvic and abdominal cavities. Eventually, it damages the tissues it comes in contact with and leads to SCAR TISSUE formation.

SYMPTOMS

Scar tissue often results in INFERTILITY or difficulty getting pregnant and endometriosis accounts for a third of this.

Scar tissue often results in CHRONIC PELVIC PAIN or pelvic pain that has persisted at least for 6 months. Most chronic pelvic pain is not gynecological though endometriosis accounts for 71 to 87% that is. Interestingly, the degree of pain is quite variable with some women experiencing severe pain from a small amount of endometriosis and others experiencing none from a lot. Endometriosis has even been found in women undergoing surgical sterilization who never complained of pain.

Scar tissue often results in DYSPAREUNIA or pain during sex.

PRESSURE often results from your enlarging uterus that is accumulating blood in its outer muscle layer.

DYSMENORRHEA or periods that are excruciatingly painful is common if your outer uterus has a lot of scar tissue or if blood has accumulated in its muscle layer.

DIAGNOSIS

THE BEST WAY TO DIAGNOSE ENDOMETRIOSIS IS LAPAROSCOPY, **which introduces a telescope through a tiny incision just under your belly button and an operating rod through a smaller one above your bladder bone.** Your pelvic and abdominal cavities are carefully scanned for anything that does not resemble the usual smooth pink shiny peritoneal lining (see Sex Organ Chapter). Endometriosis can look like scar tissue, smears of chocolate-like old blood, gunpowder burns or even clear teardrops so it is important that your surgeon has a lot of experience with all of its different forms. The operating rod is used to biopsy any suspicious areas, which are subsequently viewed under a microscope. Care must be taken not to puncture your internal organs and/or major blood vessels and there is also the risk of anesthesia.

Generally, it is performed if you have infertility or still have pain after a trial of the pill and/or Lupron. Most endometriosis is never confirmed this way however, since it costs thousands of dollars and is associated with the risks above.

COLONOSCOPY introduces a telescope into your rectum and lower colon and is generally indicated if your pain is mostly on the lower left side, have pain during a bowel movement, rectal bleeding and constipation.

CYSTOSCOPY introduces a telescope into your bladder and lower ureters and is generally indicated if you have blood in your urine and/or bladder spasms.

RECTOVAGINAL EXAM sometimes reveals nodules behind your cervix or your uterus might be tilted backwards, but unable to move from scar tissue behind it since endometriosis tends to gravitate to the bottom of your pelvis and concentrate there.

SONOGRAM, CT AND/OR MRI scans are never definite for endometriosis since they only show you contrasting shades of black, white and gray that a trained eye can hopefully interpret. Contrary to popular belief, they are not TV pictures.

This limitation aside, they may reveal an enlarged uterus and/or ovary as a result of blood accumulating inside your underlying uterine muscle layer or outside on the outer surface of your ovaries.

A finding of an enlarged ovary should trigger an additional CA-125 blood test for ovarian cancer. Unfortunately, this test was designed to follow the response of already-known ovarian cancer to chemotherapy, not to diagnose it. Consequently, it misses some ovarian cancers while also mistaking non-cancerous conditions like endometriosis and/or fibroids for it.

AS A SIDE POINT, YOU SHOULD ALSO HAVE A HYSTEROSCOPY or telescope introduced into your cervical canal and uterine cavity if you have pain since 30% have fibroids, polyps and/or cervical stenosis, which is scar tissue blocking your cervical canal and/or its opening.

ADENOMYOSIS IS DIAGNOSED ONLY AFTER HYSTERECTOMY or surgical removal of your uterus though at times an expensive MRI scan will detect lining imbedded inside your underlying muscle layer.

CLASSIFICATION

Endometriosis is classified as MINIMUM, MILD, MODERATE OR SEVERE according to its degree of spread to your ovaries, tubes, pouch-like area behind and below your uterus and remaining peritoneum.

ENDOMETRIOMAS or endometrial implants are classified as being deep or superficial and are measured in centimeters (cms).

SCAR TISSUE is classified as being filmy or dense and whether or not the affected organ is partially or completely encased.

SURGICAL TREATMENT

ELECTRIC HEAT OR LIGHT LASER BURNS THROUGH scar tissue and/or endometriomas <1 cm at the time of laparoscopy if your endometriois is minimun or mild and you have pain and/or infertility. Controversy exists over whether or not to burn your endometriosis if it is minimum or mild, you do not have pain and are not trying to get pregnant because 90% of you eventually get pregnant on your own and surgery could lead to infection and/or new scar tissue over the raw burn areas.

LAPAROTOMY or a longer abdominal incision that actually lets you touch the organs is the treatment for endometriomas >2 cms as well as moderate and severe disease. You have a 60% chance of getting pregnant if your endometriosis is moderate, but only 35 % if it is severe. Bleeding is an additional risk as well as infection. More care must be taken not to leave large exposed areas that could form new scar tissue and to avoid bowel, ureter and bladder injury. Most of the time it is done right after your laparoscopy though sometimes it is postponed for 2 to 3 months if you have particularly dense implants that require hormones to soften them up for easier removal.

THE ONLY REAL CURE IS RADICAL SURGERY that removes your uterus, tubes, ovaries and any other implants when your pain is unbearable and you no longer desire pregnancy. We give you hormones afterwards, though sometimes we leave an ovary in if it is normal and all of your other endometriosis has been removed.

HORMONAL TREATMENT

Since laparoscopy has surgical risks and is quite expensive, a 3-month trial of hormones are often given if you have pain, dyspareunia, dysmeorrhea and/or pressure that is presumed to be due to endometriosis. If your symptoms improve, your diagnosis of endometriosis has been confirmed and they are continued for at least another 3 months. Of course, if you do not improve the next step is laparoscopy to hopefully determine why not.

We also offer hormones if laparoscopy reveals minimum or mild endometriosis, but you do not have symptoms and are not trying to get pregnant in hopes of keeping it from worsening over time.

As mentioned above, hormones are sometimes given prior to laparotomy if your implants are very dense or after laparotomy for severe disease to improve your dismal 35% pregnancy rate. The latter is controversial however, since you are more likely to get pregnant occur within a year of surgery and 3 to 6 months of hormone treatment significantly cuts into this.

PROGESTERONE slows down your lining growth in response to estrogen. We usually give you a high-dose of Provera 30mg nightly or Megace or Megestrol acetate 40mg nightly for 6 months if you are trying get pregnant or Depo-Provera shots every 3 months if you are not. If water retention and depression are a problem, we drop the Provera dose to 10 or 20mg nightly or substitute Aygestin /Norethindrone acetate 5mg nightly. If irregular bleeding is a problem, we give you a week estrogen in the form Premarin 1.25mg daily or Estrace 2mg daily to build up and stabilize your lining.

CONTINUOUS COMBINED PILLS also slow down lining growth because the progesterone in them is always stronger than the estrogen. For 6 months a fresh pack is started every 21 days to avoid the monthly pill-period that occurs with regular 28-day packs. Irregular bleeding can be a problem and, again, this is treated with a week of extra estrogen or by taking it the regular way with a fresh pack every 28 days.

DANAZOL slows down lining growth by decreasing both ovarian hormones with 400mg, 600mg or 800mg a day being prescribed for 6 months. It is quite expensive and is a male-like androgen hormone, which has worse side effects like an increase in facial and body hair, acne, baldness, irreversible lowering of your voice, breast tissue shrinkage and a unfavorable cholesterol pattern that predisposes to heart attack. Water retention is often worse as well and you can also end up with hot flushes and vaginal dryness. Danazol's high cost and side effects make long-term treatment impractical though a vaginal preparation may be in the works to lessen them. Pregnancy is possible with genital birth defects sometimes occurring in female newborns.

LUPRON shots every month or every 3 months up to 6 months also decrease both ovarian hormones. It costs about $350 for 3 months and can be given at any time as long as you are not already pregnant. Though rare, pregnancy can a few weeks after your first shot since Lupron sometimes makes you ovulate initially instead of shutting down your ovaries immediately. Hot flushes and vaginal dryness are quite problematic as well as bone loss, so small amounts of estrogen and progesterone are usually added after the third month. Although it is generally too expensive for longer-term use, some women who can afford it do so.

RECURRENCE

ENDOMETRIOSIS IS BOUND TO COME BACK as long as your ovaries are making estrogen. To offset this, you should really consider long-term use of the pill or Depo-Provera if you are not trying to get pregnant versus 200mg Promethium or 10mg Provera for 10 to 14 nights each month if you are.

9

Ovarian Cysts

Since a CYST is a sac of fluid, ovarian cysts are sacs of fluid inside the ovary.

Unfortunately, there is whole lot of confusion over them since so many of you think they are something to worry about. Ladies, let me put your minds at ease and let you in on another secret. You make two cysts inside one of your ovaries one month and two more inside your other ovary the next month and so on and so on as long as you are menstruating. This is considered a normal female body event since billions of other women all over the world do the same thing each and every month!

FUNCTIONAL cysts produce your eggs while cranking out sex hormones essential to your menstrual cycle and 99.9% of ovarian cysts fall into this category.

Less than 0.01% of them are NON-FUNCTIONAL as discussed later on.

FUNTIONAL CYSTS

Again, there are two types of FUNCTIONAL or physiological ovarian cysts that you make inside one of your other ovaries one month and your other ovary the next month.

A FOLLICULAR CYST produces a follicle or egg while also cranking out estrogen sex hormone that prepares your uterine lining for a potential pregnancy. You start making this cyst on Day 1 of your period and it lasts for 10 to 14 days. It starts out microscopic in size and gradually enlarges to the size of your thumbnail so symptoms are virtually unheard of with it.

Every month around Day 15 your follicular cyst ruptures in order to release your follicle in a process called, OVULATION. This is a normal event tolerated by 99.9% of billions of women the world over despite its mild discomfort. Once in a while ovulation triggers significant bleeding, but generally this is limited to those of you with bleeding disorders. This could result in significant pain as well as life-saving surgery to control the bleeding.

An OVULATORY CYST forms as your follicular cyst heals over, accumulates more fluid and produce progesterone sex hormone along with more estrogen to further prepare your lining. This cyst lasts for 9 to 11 days and often causes a throbbing sensation a few days right before your period when it has reached its maximum size. A lot of you think you can feel it with your own hands, but this is impossible since it is only as big as a ping-pong ball and sinks behind your uterus.

An ovulatory cyst rarely ruptures, but when it does you can also have significant bleeding because it has an extensive network of blood vessels. Again, severe pain may result and surgery is generally required.

Both hormone levels plummet around Day 25 when your ovulatory cyst dies if no sperm has united with your egg within 24 hours of its release and there is no resultant pregnancy hormone around to keep it alive.

Your prepared lining starves, dies and is sloughed off as a period around Day 28. At the same time, a new follicular cyst forms on your other ovary while your body re-absorbs the fluid in your ovulatory cyst, which disappears a few days later.

DIAGNOSIS

Most functional cysts are diagnosed after they are felt on a BIMANUAL EXAM. An enlarged ovary felt 14 days or less after the onset of your period is generally assumed to be a follicular cyst. An enlarged ovary felt 15 days or more after the onset of your period is generally assumed to be an ovulatory cyst. If your periods are irregular or absent and both ovaries are enlarged, they may be POLYCYSTIC or contain multiple small cysts clustered along their edges (see Amenorrhea Chapter).

Many cysts are also picked up by a PELVIC SONOGRAM, which bounces sound waves off fluid-filled structures.

TRANSABDOMINAL pelvic sonograms are performed by pressing a sound wave device over your urine-filled bladder, which helps these waves travel to your internal organs and back again. Unfortunately, there is considerable distance between the device and your ovaries, which are often difficult to see if your bowel is full of gas and stool, swollen and/or stuck together.

TRANSVAGINAL pelvic sonograms do not require a full bladder. The sound wave device is closer to your ovaries so there is less bowel interference, however. Of course, having that device in between your legs is a little awkward.

The images that are obtained from either are simply shades of black, white and gray that a trained eye can interpret. They are not TV pictures, however.

Beware of medical professionals who tell you that you have a "ruptured cyst" just because fluid is seen on your pelvic sonogram. Your pelvic and abdominal cavities are always moist with fluid that is supposed to be seen on a pelvic sonogram. The amount of fluid that is released from your thumbnail-sized follicular cyst at ovulation is negligible compared to this.

TREATMENT

Functional cysts rarely require treatment since your body reabsorbs the fluid in them every month. Again, you may need surgery if you bleed significantly at ovulation or if your ovulatory cyst ruptures.

Occasionally, we give combined pills or Depo-Provera if you have a bleeding disorder or if your cysts are consistently symptomatic and/or excessively large. Combined pills keep you from making any new cysts and Depo-Provera lets you make only small follicular cysts that do not progress to ovulation.

NON-FUNCTIONAL CYSTS

NON-FUNCTIONAL **or pathological ovarian cysts occur in 0.1% of all women.** A full discussion of them is beyond the scope of this handout, but I have provided a few details below.

Most are not cancerous, but this obviously worries us the most since ovarian cancer tends to be advanced when discovered.

We suspect them if we feel a mass a few days after your period starts or 1 or 2 months after you have been on combined pills or Depo-Provera.

We suspect them anytime we feel your ovary after menopause because they are normally the size of a shelled almond and are too small to feel.

We suspect them if your ovary is larger than a ping-pong and your periods are regular.

We also suspect them when they do not have the characteristic appearance of a functional cyst on your sonogram.

You may need X-RAYS, CT and/or MRI scans if there is an uncharacteristic appearance, especially if ovarian cancer is suspected and to see if it has spread.

Sometimes we send a Ca-125 ovarian cancer blood test, but this misses some ovarian cancers. Also, non-cancerous conditions like fibroids and endometriosis often give high results that are often mistaken for cancer. This test was originally designed to follow your response to chemotherapy for documented ovarian cancer and is obviously not 100% accurate at picking it up. There are other cancer blood tests like CEA, AFP and HCG that may be sent as well.

Most require surgery to obtain a definite diagnosis, but a few do not if their appearance suggests a non-functional cyst that is not cancerous.

LAPAROSCOPY introduces a telescope through a tiny incision under your belly button and an operating rod through a smaller one just above your bladder bone. This does provide a TV picture of your ovaries and other internal organs. We generally perform it when your cyst is smaller than your uterus and when cancer is not suspected. Sometimes your cyst is drained and a small portion of it is biopsied or removed for tissue analysis under a microscope. Occasionally, it can even be removed, with or without your ovary.

EXPLORATORY LAPAROTOMY is more extensive surgery through a larger incision to allow direct contact with your organs. We generally perform this when your cyst is larger than your uterus or when cancer is suspected and all of your other pelvic organs need to be removed as well.

TREATMENT DEPENDS ON THE TYPE OF NON-FUNCTIONAL CYST and ranges from observation over time, surgical removal via laparoscopy and/or exploratory laparotomy, chemotherapy and/or radiation.

10

Fibroids

Most all of you are familiar with fibroids, which are BENIGN TUMORS or non-cancerous new growths located in the outer muscle layer of your uterus and cervix. They are also called, "Myomas" or "Leiomyomatas" and <1 in 1,000 are cancerous.

Specifically speaking, they are muscle cells that feed off your hormones and grow in response to them.

Estrogen definitely makes them grow though progesterone has mixed effects. Fortunately, it usually shrinks far more fibroids than it grows.

They grow progressively from your first period to your last or as long as your ovaries are making hormones from puberty to menopause.

They are more common in obese women since they make more estrogen than thin ones from fat cells that change other hormones into extra estrogen.

They are 2 to 3 times more common in black women for unclear reasons though more of them are obese with a possible genetic component as well.

They are usually multiple with fibroids present in varying sizes and locations throughout your uterus and cervix though a few predominate in size and symptoms.

SYMPTOMS

Though 50% of NON-PREGNANT women never have symptoms from their fibroids, the other half often experience:

1. **MENORRHAGIA or heavy periods** since they increase the overall size of your uterus, its inner cavity and the lining you slough off as a period.
2. **MENOMETRORRHAGIA or irregular and/or heavy bleeding when they DEGENERATE AND/OR ABORT.** Fibroids degenerate or decompose when they greedily grow faster than their blood supply. Fibroids on the end of a long stalk can abort or be painfully delivered through your cervix like a pregnancy.
3. **DYSMENORRHEA or excruciatingly painful periods** from normal muscle having to squeeze harder around fibroids and to push out more lining than usual.
4. **DYSPAREUNIA or pain during sex.**
5. **Pain unrelated to the menstrual cycle** when the uterus flops around as a result of being attached to a pair of stretched-out broad ligaments. Degenerating and/or aborting fibroids also cause the same type of pain.
6. **Pressure on the bladder and/or rectum,** which results in frequent urination, bladder control difficulties and/or constipation.
7. **Sagging of the vagina, bladder and/or rectum** due to the effect of gravity on a heavier than usual uterus.
8. **Difficulty getting pregnant.**

Though 33% of PREGNANT women improve and another 33% have no change in their fibroids, the remaining 33% often experience:

1. **Miscarriage** before the 20th week of pregnancy.
2. **Degeneration with pain so severe** that a prolonged hospital stay is required for narcotic pain injections medication.
3. **Premature labor and delivery after the 20th week of pregnancy,** especially if they cause your membranes to rupture.
4. **A Cesarean section** if they make your labor inefficient and/or block your birth canal.
5. **Excessive blood loss at delivery.**

DIAGNOSIS

More than 25% of you have fibroids that are diagnosed in your 30's or 40's when they are generally large enough to cause symptoms and/or be detected. These fibroids no doubt existed years earlier, but were too small to be noticed.

Many fibroids are felt during the BIMANUAL portion of your pelvic exam.

Others are detected on a PELVIC SONOGRAM, which bounces sound waves off fluid-filled structures.

TRANSABDOMINAL pelvic sonograms are performed by pressing a sound wave device over your urine-filled bladder, which helps these waves travel to your internal organs and back again. Unfortunately, there is considerable distance between the device and your internal sex organs with small fibroids often being difficult to see if your bowel is full of gas and stool, swollen and/or stuck together.

TRANSVAGINAL pelvic sonograms do not require a full bladder since the sound wave device is right up against your uterus. This makes it ideal for finding small fibroids inside your cavity. Sometimes, water is squirted inside your cavity first to make them show up even better. Of course, having the device in your vagina is a bit awkward.

The images that are obtained from either are simply shades of black, white and gray that a trained eye can interpret. They are not TV pictures, however.

A few fibroids will be noticed on a PELVIC CT AND/OR MRI SCAN.

Considerably more are seen on a PELVIC X-RAY if they are calcified.

Fewer are seen on an infertility HYSTEROSALPINGOGRAM or HSG x-ray dye test of your uterine cavity and tubes if you are having trouble conceiving.

Rarely, they may be seen during uterine, pelvic or abdominal SURGERY, particularly if the uterine cavity is bumpy during an endometrial biopsy or D+C.

At times, muscle fibers are found in an endometrial biopsy or D+C specimen.

TREATMENT

IGNORING SMALL FIBROIDS WILL HAUNT YOU IN THE FUTURE!

Growth is likely to grow even if you do not have symptoms so it is extremely important to monitor your uterine size via exam and/or sonogram every 6 months. Generally, your uterus is significantly enlarged when it is bigger than a Sunkist orange.

PROGESTERONE hormone generally slows down fibroid growth in response to estrogen, yet long-term treatment is required for years until menopause. If you desire birth control, you can try Depo-Provera shots every 3 months or even every month in you also have menorrhagia as well. If you are trying to conceive, you can try Provera 10mg or Promethium 200mg for 10 to 14 consecutive nights each month.

COMBINED PILLS also slow down fibroid growth. They contain estrogen as well as progesterone, but the progesterone is always stronger than the estrogen.

MONTHLY LUPRON SHOTS keep your ovaries from making hormones and is generally given 3 to 6 months before surgery. They are quite expensive and menopausal-like side effects are common so we usually do not give it for much longer.

ANTIBIOTICS, PAIN MEDS AND BEDREST treats degenerating fibroids, though surgery may be required if this does not work.

MYOMECTOMY or surgically removing some of your fibroids is an option if you have significant bleeding, pain and/or trouble getting pregnant. This procedure should never be taken lightly however, since it is associated with a significant risk of extreme bleeding that can result in hysterectomy or removal of your entire uterus.

IT IS A TEMPORARY FIX however, since your symptoms often return months to years later when the other fibroids that were left in grow over time!

Myomectomy is performed several ways according to location of your fibroids, your medical condition and your gynecologist's skill and familiarity with technique.

1. **Sometimes aborting fibroids are VAGINALLY removed in the office** by placing a sterile clamp on the stalk while repeatedly twisting it until it is released. Again, bleeding is a risk and an operating room is this safest place to do this.
2. **HYSTEROSCOPY is good for small fibroids that protrude into your cavity.** This same-day surgical procedure introduces a telescope inside your uterus so your fibroids can be plucked out, shaved or burned down.
3. **LAPAROSCOPY is good for small fibroids attacheed by a stalk to your uterus.** This is another same-day surgery that introduces a telescope through a tiny incision under your belly button and an operating rod through a smaller one over your

bladder bone. A loop of suture is tightened like a noose around the stalk and the fibroid is cut off or burned off above it. The fibroid is removed through the bladder incision that may have been enlarged to an inch or two or a third incision that was added on either side of your lower abdomen. Care must be taken not to injure your bowel, bladder or major blood vessels on top of your spine when introducing the telescope, however.

4. **LAPAROSCOPY is also used to apply spot burns across larger fibroids, particularly their surface blood vessels. Over time, they degenerate and decrease in size.** These spot burns are achieved by running an electric current thru a needle attached to the operating probe.
5. **ABDOMINAL LAPAROTOMY removes the most fibroids through a 6-inch** or longer incision that provides enough room to open up your uterus, pluck out several dozen fibroids and sew it back up. Again, care must be taken not to injure your bowel and bladder as well as the pair of major blood vessels that run along both sides of your cervix. This requires a 4-to 7-day hospital stay due to narcotic pain medication for your longer incision and bowel to recover from being partially paralyzed as a result of being tucked away out the operating field and narcotic pain medication needed for the longer incision.

HYSTERECTOMY or removing your entire uterus is the most effective treatment. Generally, it is performed when no more children are desired and/or when other methods have failed on a uterus larger than a grapefruit. A uterus larger than this is less likely to respond to progesterone and can potentially reverse the flow of urine up into your kidneys, especially if fibroids are clustered around your cervix. The latter can result in repeated kidney infections, scarring and subsequent damage.

Hysterectomy is performed several ways as well.

1. **If your uterus is not too large, VAGINAL REMOVAL may be attempted.** We also suggest this if you have a sagging bladder

and/or rectum that also needs repair. Again, care must be taken not to injure your bladder and bowel as well as the ureters or tube to each kidney, which enters the bladder near your cervix. It has the advantage of a shorter 2-to 3-day hospital stay since you have a small vaginal incision and your bowel are not tucked away.

2. **VAGINAL REMOVAL AND LAPAROSCOPY CAN BE COMBINED** by particularly skilled surgeons. This technique is especially appropriate when there is a possibility that scar tissue will prevent vaginal removal or to get a good look at your ovaries if they were suspicious on a prior sonogram since ovarian cancer requires abdominal surgery. Again, care must be taken not to injure your bowel, bladder, ureters and major blood vessels. This has a shorter 1-to 2-day hospital stay, though if your vagina is also repaired you may need to stay 1 or 2 days more.
3. **ABDOMINAL REMOVAL is the most common technique,** especially if your uterus is large. Again, care must be takenAgain, this generally requires a longer 4-to 7-day hospital stay.

Part III

Infection Topics

11

Yeast

Yeast—also called "Candida" or "Monilia"—is in the fungus class of germ organisms.

LADIES, YOU DO NOT GET YEAST FROM EATING BREAD!

A different kind of Yeast is normally found in small amounts all over your skin, inside your digestive tract from your mouth to your anus, your vagina and your cervix. When the environment changes, it can overgrow and invade your underlying tissues to cause inflammation and a true infection.

This Yeast prefers dark, warm, moist, sweet areas that are frequently exposed to sweat and/or moisture, yet unexposed to light or fresh circulating air like the:

Vagina	Foot soles
Cervix	Armpits
Vulva or outer genital lips	Skin underneath both breasts
Upper thigh-hip skin folds	Skin underneath an overhanging belly

GENITAL INFECTION SITES

In women, the genital areas infected by Yeast include your **vagina, cervix, vulva, perineum and urethra.**

PREDISPOSING FACTORS

Yeast is common if you DOUCHE, since this washes away the good organisms that normally keep it in check. Vinegar douching is virtually a recipe for Yeast.

Yeast is common if you are taking ANTIBIOTICS since they kill the good organisms that normally keep it in check.

Yeast is common if you are DIABETIC because you have a lot of sugar in your bloodstream.

Yeast is common if you are OBESE and/or PREGNANT because you have unexposed skin folds and are prone to have a lot of sugar as well.

Yeast is common if you are taking STEROIDS that weaken your immune system like Prednisone, Hydrocortisone and Lidex creams, Vancenase and Beclonase inhalers.

Yeast is common if your immune system is weak from HIV and/or CANCER, especially if you had chemotherapy and/or radiation therapy.

SYMPTOMS

You can have NO SYMPTOMS or any of the following.

1. **Itching, burning, redness and/or swelling** of your vulva and vagina that frequently causes pain during sex.
2. **Cottage cheese or a curd-like discharge or an increase in your usual** creamy white discharge.
3. **Pain when you urinate and/or frequent urination.**

None of these symptoms are unique to Yeast since they also occur with other infections and conditions. For instance, itching and burning is also common when you have Trichomonas and/or DIV, a little-known, relatively new, hard-to-diagnose bacterial infection (see both of these chapters). Also, an increase in your usual creamy white discharge is also seen in BV, another well known easy to diagnose bacterial infection (see this chapter also).

DIAGNOSIS

A SALINE PREP MICROSCOPIC VAGINAL DISCHARGE EXAM **is the quickest, cheapest, most common and most accurate way to diagnose Yeast.** We simply place a tiny bit of your discharge on a rectangular glass slide, mix it with a drop of salt water and cover it with a smaller thinner glass square. Next, we place it under a microscope in the office, clinic and/or ER and check it for various Yeast forms, other organisms, inflammatory white cells and/or sperm right after finishing your pelvic.

You should SPECIFICALLY REQUEST a saline prep if you have itching and/or a lot of discharge, especially if your vulva, vagina and/or cervix appear irritated. It should even be considered when your discharge, vulva, vagina and/or cervix all appear normal and pink in order to exclude an early infection that has not had time to fully set in.

Of course, your saline prep is more accurate when it is performed regularly by your medical professional rather than once in a while since practice makes perfect.

Beware of medical professionals who rely on the appearance of your discharge and/or PAP smear result alone! I cannot tell you how many times I was fooled into thinking that Yeast always looked like cottage cheese or that Trichomonas always had to be frothy yellow only to be proved wrong under the microscope. The PAP was designed for cancer and the changes that occur before this, not infection. As a result, it misses far more infections than it ever picks up! It also takes 5 to 14 days to come back.

A saline prep is impossible to interpret during your period when blood replaces most of your discharge.

It is difficult to interpret after you douche your discharge away.

It is difficult to interpret when you have more than one infection.

It is extremely difficult to interpret if you have any medication in your vagina that is mixed in with your discharge. This usually happens if you after incorrectly assuming that Yeast is the cause of your symptoms and use an over-the-counter (OTC) anti-fungal medication without having an exam to confirm it.

Although Yeast can be MENTIONED ON YOUR PAP REPORT, this does not mean that you have an infection since it is normally found inside your vagina and cervix.

If your infection persists, your Yeast can be CULTURED IN A SPECIAL GEL designed to grow fungus. This confirms that you have Yeast, identifies what type of Yeast you have and determines which anti-fungal treatment is most effective.

We often test you for Gonorrhea and Chlamydia (see both of these chapters) because they both cause a lot of discharge and/or an irritated cervix, but are not seen under the microscope.

TREATMENT

Vaginal cream, suppositories and inserts work the best and are used at night while you are lying down flat for a few hours. They may be messy, but it is important to complete the entire 3-or 7-night course even if you feel better before. If your period interrupts this, resume it after. If your outer genital skin is infected, you need to apply cream twice a day for 1 to 2 weeks and even swallow oral tablets as well if it is severe.

Prescription (Rx) preparations are:

1. **Terconazole**/Terazol-3 is the most effective and comes as a 3-night course of 80mg vaginal suppositories and 0.8% cream. Terazol-7 is half as concentrated at 0.4% and comes only as a 7-night cream.
2. **Fluconazole**/Diflucan one-dose 150mg oral tablet works best if you are on your period or have to wear skimpy costumes or a bathing suit. If your infection is particularly severe, we sometimes give you 100mg or 200mg tablets once or twice daily for 1 to 2 weeks.
3. **Clotrimazole**/Mycelex-G comes as a one-dose 500mg vaginal tablet and 1% cream that is applied once or twice day for 1 to 2 weeks. There is also a Twin Pack that combines both of these.
4. **Miconazole**/Monistat-3 comes as a 3-night course of 200mg vaginal suppositories and a Dual Pak with a one-dose 1200mg vaginal suppository as well as a 2% cream that is applied once or twice a day for 1 to 2 weeks.
5. **Butaconazole**/Gynazole-1 comes as a one-night 2% vaginal cream that actually hangs around for 4 days.
6. **Mycostatin**/Nystatin comes in the form of 100,000Units/gram vaginal tablet, cream and powder that are all used for 2 weeks.
7. **Ketoconazole**/Nizoral comes in the form of a 200mg oral tablet that is taken once daily for several months if your infection is persistent.
8. **Boric acid** in the form of a 600mg capsule can be placed in your vagina at bedtime for 2 weeks for persistent infection as well. Yes, this also kills roaches.

OTC non-prescription preparations are:

1. **Tioconazole**/Vagistat-1 and Monistat-1 are different brand names for the same one-night 6.5% vaginal ointment that hangs around for 3 nights.

2. **Butaconazole**/Femstat-3 and Mycelex-3 are different brand names for the same 3-night 2% vaginal cream.
3. **Miconazole**/Monistat-3 Combination Pack consists of a 2% cream that is applied once or twice daily for 1 to 2 weeks and a 3-night course of 200mg vaginal suppositories, Monistat-7 comes as a 2% cream and 100mg vaginal suppositories as well as a Combination Pack that contains both and Lotrimin-AF 2% comes as a spray and powder.
4. **Clotrimazole**/Mycelex-7 and Gyne-Lotrimin are different brand names for the same 7-night course of 100mg vaginal tablets, 1% cream and Combination Pack, Gyne-Lotrimin 3 comes as a 3-night course of 200mg vaginal tablets and a Combination-Pack that also has a 1% cream and both Lotrimin and Desenex come in the form of a 1% cream, solution and powder.
5. **Tolnaftate**/Tinactin comes in the form of a 1% cream, powder, solution or spray.

Other treatments include:

1. **Controlling your blood sugar** through diet and diabetic medications.
2. **Controlling your weight** through diet and exercise.
3. **Not suffocating your vaginal opening** with multiple clothes layers.
4. **Maintaining a clean shower surface** and drying your toes immediately.
5. **Consider a preventative one-dose anti-fungal** when you take antibiotics.
6. **Anti-retroviral HIV medications.**

If you have itching and burning yet bleeding prevents a saline prep, we often give you a trial of Metronidazole 2g for possible Trichomonas along with Diflucan 150mg for possible Yeast as well.

If you still have no relief and have abstained from sex, you could have DIV and may need an additional 6-to 7-night course of Clindamycin/Cleocin 2% vaginal cream and/or suppository-ovules when you stop bleeding to treat this.

Although Lactobacilli bacteria keep Yeast in check, it is impossible to re-stock your vagina with it by eating yogurt or drinking it from a bottle since neither contains enough live bacteria to be effective.

You should probably avoid sex during your treatment for Yeast to keep as much medication as possible in your vagina and to give it chance to heal.

Although it cannot be proved that Yeast is passed from person-to-person during sex since everyone has it, persistent episodes often resolve after treating your partner.

OTC Yeast-Gard (which actually contains Yeast!), Vagi-Gard, Vagisil, Vaginex, Vagicaine, Benzocaine, A+D, Summer's Eve Medicated Anti-Itch, Gynecort, Hydrocortisone, Cortaid and Cortisone are not anti-fungals so they WILL NOT TREAT YEAST, only make it worse!

DOUCHING

There is nothing that gets me going more than the subject of douching!

Douching, feminine deodorants and powders never clean you, so they are not recommended for routine hygiene, odor or increased discharge!

Douching only puts money in the pockets of men who do not! Just because you can buy them, do not assume that they are good for you, as the deceptive advertising would have you believe. You can also buy alcohol and cigarettes, but neither is good for you!

Douching for odor and/or increased discharge is like a dog chasing its own tail since it causes BV and/or Yeast infections by washing away the good organisms that keep the bad ones in check. While douching may temporarily relieve your symptoms, it does not get at the root of your problem or the infection itself. The infection continues to produce the odor and/or increased discharge that makes you douche over and over again!

Douching causes more serious pelvic infections involving the uterus, tubes and ovaries, particularly if you do it after your period. During your period the opening to your uterus is wider than usual to let your blood flow out. Since blood is good food for the smaller amounts of bacteria that are normally present, their numbers subsequently increase. Douching after your period only flushes this nasty bacterial soup up inside your uterus.

12

Trichomonas

Trichomonas—also called "Trick" (or my favorite, "Tricky Dick")—is in the parasite class of germ organisms.

TRANSMISSION

Trichomonas is a STD or SEXUALLY-TRANSMITTED DISEASE that is passed from person-to-person through close intimate sexual contact, including acts other than vaginal-penile penetration. This includes female-to-female sex as well as so-called virgins who engage in "heavy petting" without actually being penetrated!

TRANSLATION: He doesn't have to stick it in for you to get it! Just having his penis in the vicinity of the outside vulva and vaginal orifice is enough for you to get it!

You can also pass it on to your newborn's mouth and throat during birth. This can lead to excessive crying and poor feeding during the first few weeks of life.

In rare cases you can get it from a warm soiled towel, underwear or bathing suit that has just been used by someone else, but if you do this you are probable having sex with that person. You cannot get Trichomonas from soiled towels, underwear or bathing suits that have been sitting around for a while, a moist toilet seat, steam room, sauna, jacuzzi, hot tub or pool.

INFECTION SITES

Trichomonas infects your **vagina, cervix, vulva, urethra, perineum, mouth and throat.**

SYMPTOMS

You can have NO SYMPTOMS or any of the following.

1. **Itching, burning, redness and/or swelling** of your vulva and vagina that frequently causes pain during sex.
2. **Yellow frothy vaginal discharge that frequently has an odor or an increase** in your usual creamy white discharge.
3. **Pain when you urinate and/or frequent urination.**
4. **Sore throat** along with an irritating cough.

Again, none of these symptoms are unique to Trichomonas since they also occur with other infections and conditions. For instance, itching and burning is also common when you have Yeast and DIV, a little-known, relatively new, hard-to-diagnose bacterial infection (see both of these chapters).

DIAGNOSIS

AGAIN, A SALINE PREP MICROSCOPIC VAGINAL DISCHARGE EXAM is the quickest, cheapest and most common way to diagnose Trichomonas. This is explained in detail in the Yeast Chapter.

It is 80 to 90% accurate if you have symptoms and/or irritation since the Trichomonad organisms are usually moving then. This drops to only 50 to 60% however, when you do not since they are usually not moving then. Since it is so hard to diagnose Trichomonas accurately, it is not unusual to offer treatment for it even if there are no moving organisms on the saline prep.

Again, it is difficult to interpret your saline prep during your period, after you douche, if you have more than one infection or after mistakenly inserting an over-the-counter (OTC) Yeast medication.

Again, you should SPECIFICALLY REQUEST a saline prep if you have itching and/or a lot of discharge, especially if your vulva, vagina and/or cervix appear irritated. It should even be considered when your discharge, vulva, vagina and/or cervix all appear normal pink to exclude an early infection that has not had a chance to cause a lot of discharge and irritation yet.

Again, your saline prep is more accurate when it is performed regularly by your medical professional rather than once in a while since practice makes perfect.

Again, beware of medical professionals who rely on the appearance of your discharge and/or PAP smear result alone! I cannot tell you how many times I was fooled into thinking that Yeast always looked like cottage cheese or that Trichomonas always had to be frothy yellow only to be proved wrong under the microscope. The PAP was designed for precancerous and cancerous cervical changes, not infection so it misses far more of them than it ever picks up! It also takes 5 to 14 days for your results to come back.

Even so, Trichomonas is sometimes MENTIONED ON YOUR PAP REPORT.

Trichomonas can also be CULTURED IN A SPECIAL BROTH designed to grow parasites. However, this is time-consuming since it takes 3 to 7 days and expensive.

Sometimes a MICROSCOPIC URINE EXAM will detect moving organisms if you have urinary symptoms and/or an irritated urethral meatus.

We rarely send DNA or ANTIBODY tests that detect substances that your body makes in response to Chlamydia since they are also expensive.

Again, we often test you for Gonorrhea and Chlamydia (see both of these chapters) because they also cause a lot of discharge and/or an irritated cervix, but are not seen easily under the microscope.

A lot of you look at me like I am stark raving mad when I tell you that you have a STD, yet you have not had sex for a while. I hate to burst your bubble, but mad I am not.

STD'S DO NOT GO AWAY JUST BECAUSE YOU STOP HAVING SEX!

You get STD's from sex, but the opposite is not true. An STD like Trichomonas is more than happy to live inside you until you die—with or without sex—since your body supplies everything it needs to survive!

TREATMENT

THE ONLY TREATMENT FOR TRICHOMONAS IS METRONIDAZOLE, which is brand-named Flagyl or Protostat. We usually give you 2 grams to take by mouth all at once or split into two separate 1-gram doses twelve hours apart or even four 500mg doses 6 hours apart. Occasionally, we give you a larger dose over a longer course of time if you have a rare resistant strain.

The uncoated tablet has a very downright nasty metallic after-taste and frequently nauseates you or even makes you vomit, particularly if you drink alcohol. I recommend that you take it an hour after a meal with a thick syrupy liquid like peach or pear nectar. Crushing it up and mixing it into pudding or applesauce does not improve its taste.

Coated Flagyl 375 gel capsules are better tolerated, but more expensive. We usually prescribed them twice daily for a week.

Metronidazole does not cause birth defects in humans and can be used if you are pregnant, especially since Trichomonas has been linked to premature labor.

MetroGel-Vaginal 0.75% or Metronidazole gel does not kill Trichomonas since it is not strong enough. If used, it should be combined with oral tablets.

Intravenous Metronidazole is reserved for more serious pelvic infections or if you cannot tolerate oral tablets despite anti-vomiting medication.

True allergic reactions are virtually non-existent.

You may need a lower dose if you are on Coumadin/Warfarin blood thinner or have a bad liver or bad kidneys.

You should consider using a one-night OTC anti-fungal since Metronidazole is also an antibiotic and might cause an overgrowth of Yeast.

If your symptoms persist despite treatment and abstinence, you could have DIV and may need Cleocin/Clindamycin-2% vaginal cream and/or suppository-ovules for 6 to 7 nights to treat it.

If you have itching and burning yet bleeding prevents a saline prep, we often give you a simple trial of one-dose Metronidazole 2g and Fluconazole 150mg to cover Trichomonas as well asYeast.

Prescription Sultrin cream, OTC anti-fungals and other anti-itch preparations like A+D, Vagisil, Vaginex, Vagicaine, Benzocaine, Lanicaine, Summer's Eve Medicated, Gynecort, Hydrocortisone, Cortaid and Cortisone WILL NOT TREAT TRICHOMONAS, only make it worse!

DOUCHING

You may recognize this same Douching Section from the previous Yeast Chapter, but I feel compelled to repeat it a second time since this is such a destructive habit!

Douching, feminine deodorants and powders never clean you so they are not recommended for routine hygiene, odor or increased discharge!

Douching only puts money in the pockets of men who do not! Do not assume that being able to purchase them makes them good for you, as the deceptive advertising would have you believe. You can also buy alcohol and cigarettes, but they aren't good for you either!

Douching for odor and/or increased discharge is like a dog chasing it's own tail since it causes BV and Yeast infections that produce both symptoms by washing away your good organisms that keep your bad ones in check. While douching may temporarily relieve your symptoms, it does not get at the root of your problem, the infection itself. The infection continues to produce the odor and/or increased discharge that makes you douche over and over again!

Douching causes more serious pelvic infections involving your uterus, tubes and ovaries, particularly if you do it after your period. During your period the opening to your uterus is wider than usual to let your blood flow out. Your blood is good food for the smaller amounts of bacteria that are normally present so their numbers subsequently increase. Douching after your period flushes this nasty bacterial soup up inside your uterus.

MALE INFECTION

Since Trichomonas is a STD, it would be criminal not to arm you with information about this infection in men!

It primarily INFECTS their much longer penile urethra. Rarely, Trichomonas infects their PROSTATE or the walnut-sized structure encircling their urethra where it emerges from their bladder that provides the non-sperm portion of semen and their EPIDIDYMIS or the coiled sac on top of their TESTICLES or balls where sperm mature and gain the ability to move.

Usually, they have NO SYMPTOMS or urinary ones if present.

IT IS ALMOST IMPOSSIBLE TO DETECT since a saline prep cannot be done due to a lack of penile discharge, which is washed away every time he urinates.

While it is possible to get discharge from the prostate, this is difficult to do since it requires a prolonged 5-minute rectal exam to massage the neighboring prostate, which is usually quite tender. Then it takes another 20 minutes for its milky discharge to finally appear at the tip of the penis. When it does, the prostate discharge it is similarly examined under a microscope by an Urologist, preferably. Again, this is the best type of medical professional to perform this tedious test since practice makes perfect.

Unfortunately, Trichomonas is often mistaken for Chlamydia whenever men report burning during urination, frequent urination and/or a penile discharge, yet a negative Gonorrhea test result. After being correctly diagnosed with "NGU" or Non-Gonococcal Urethritis, they are incorrectly treated for Chlamydia by many medical professionals who fail to test for it even though there are several other infections that cause the same symptoms!

Your male partner needs to specifically say, "My partner has Trichomonas" as opposed to vague stuff like "My girl said I gave her an infection." This only sends the medical professional on a wild goose chase and more often than not results in a missed diagnosis since there are many types of infections. There is no need for the medical professional to be tortured with a game of "Twenty Questions" when they are simply trying to help!

Do not be surprised if your partner tells you no testing was done at all since it is still quite common for a lot of medical professionals to just write out a Metronidazole prescription!

Again, Metronidazole is the sole treatment for Trichomonas, though larger doses and longer courses are required along with an additional antibiotic for prostatitis and/or epididymitis because multiple bacteria are also involved.

Your partner should be treated 48 hours or more before you resume sex or your treatment will be wasted!

Do not be surprised if you are given a double-dose of Metronidazole to share with your partner, though you should encourage him or her to seek separate testing and treatment. Make sure you question your partner about medication allergies, blood thinner medications, liver and/or kidney disease before giving it, however.

Being treated once will not keep you from getting it again from your same or a new one! You can almost expect to get Trichomonas with every new partner since I see it in 50% to 75% of my female patients and that many men have it, if not more!

Sad to say, I have had Trichomonas several times! I was not born a gynecologist, you know. There was a time when I too was young and stupid. Since I also had to pick up 2 other STD's before I got smart, do not follow my example!

Use barrier protection to lower your chances of infection!

13

Bacterial Vaginosis

Bacterial Vaginosis—also called "BV"—is obviously in the bacterial class of germ organisms.

BV is an overgrowth of bacteria germ organisms. Like Yeast, small amounts of bacteria normally live inside your vagina. Like Yeast, when the environment is changed, bacteria can grow too much. Like Yeast, douching often leads to BV.

Specifically, ANAEROBIC or air-hating bacteria grow too much and not the AEROBIC or air-loving ones.

BV is no longer called, "Non-specific Vagintis" or "Gardnerella" since the type of bacteria responsible for BV are specifically known without Gardnerella being one of them.

COMPLICATIONS

BV increases your risk of a serious pelvic infection after a miscarriage, vaginal delivery, voluntary abortion, Cesarean section or other pelvic surgeries.

If you are pregnant, BV increases your risk of premature labor and delivery if your membranes rupture and uterine infection as well.

SYMPTOMS

You can have NO SYMPTOMS or any of the following.

1. **Fishy odor**, particularly after sex.
2. **An increase in your usual creamy white discharge** that is often mistaken for Yeast (see this chapter).

Again, neither symptom is unique to DIV since both also occur with other infections and conditions or infections.

BV does not cause itching, burning, redness and/or swelling. If present, another infection is responsible like Trichomonas since BV frequently follows this or Yeast since it also caused by douching.

DIAGNOSIS

AGAIN, A SALINE PREP MICROSCOPIC VAGINAL DISCHARGE EXAM **is the quickest, cheapest, most common and most accurate way to diagnose BV if there are CLUE CELLS or vaginal surface cells that have lots of bacteria** all over them. This exam is explained in detail in the Yeast Chapter and there should not be any inflammatory white cells present. If they are, another infection is also present.

At times, a drop of potassium hydroxide is added for a KOH WHIFF TEST, which results in a fishy odor if BV is present.

Again, it is difficult to interpret your saline prep during your period, after you douche, if you have more than one infection or after mistakenly inserting an over-the-counter (OTC) Yeast medication.

Again, you should SPECIFICALLY REQUEST **a saline prep if you have itching and/or a lot of discharge, especially if your vulva, vagina and/or cervix appear irritated.** It should even be considered when your discharge, vulva, vagina and/or cervix all appear normal pink to exclude an early infection that has not had a chance to cause a lot of discharge and irritation yet.

Again, your saline prep is more accurate when it is performed regularly by your medical professional rather than once in a while since practice makes perfect.

Again, beware of medical professionals who rely on the appearance of your discharge and/or your PAP smear result alone! I cannot tell you how many times I was fooled into thinking that Yeast always looked like cottage cheese or that Trichomonas always had to be frothy yellow only to be proved wrong under the microscope. The PAP was designed for pre-cancerous and cancerous cervical changes, not infection so it misses far more of them than it ever picks up! It also takes 5 to 14 days for your results to come back.

Although bacteria are sometimes MENTIONED ON YOUR PAP REPORT, this does not mean that you actually have an infection since they are normally found on your vagina and cervix.

Again, CULTURING IS OF NO USE since bacteria are always present in your vagina and anaerobic bacteria are extremely difficult to grow.

Again, we often test you for Gonorrhea and Chlamydia (see both of these chapters) because they also cause a lot of discharge and are not seen easily under the microscope.

TREATMENT

We treat your BV with any of the ANTIBIOTICS below.

1. **Metronidazole / Flagyl or Protostat** tablets in a 500mg dose twice daily for a week is more effective than a one-time 2gram dose or MetroGel-Vaginal 0.75% that is inserted into your vagina at bedtime for 5 nights. The oral and intravenous forms

are more effective than the gel in preventing uterine infections if you are the pregnant. The oral form is also preferred if you have Trichomonas as well as BV. Please review the section on Metronidazole in the Trichomonas Chapter.

2. **Clindamycin / Cleocin** tablets in a 300mg dose twice daily for a week or Cleocin 2% cream and/or suppository-ovules are inserted into your vagina at bedtime for 3 nights.
3. **Amoxacillin-Clavulanic acid / Augmentin** 500mg tablet is given three times daily with meals for a week.

You should consider using a one-night OTC anti-fungal since antibiotics might cause an overgrowth of Yeast.

Although it cannot be proved that BV is passed from person-to-person during sex since everyone has bacteria, persistent episodes often resolve after treating your partner.

DOUCHING

You may recognize this same Douching Section from the Yeast Chapter, but I feel compelled to repeat it a third time since **DOUCHING IS A MAJOR CAUSE OF BV!**

Douching, feminine deodorants and powders never clean you so they are not recommended for routine hygiene, odor or increased discharge!

Douching only puts money in the pockets of men who do not! Do not assume that being able to purchase them makes them good for you, as the deceptive advertising would have you believe. You can also buy alcohol and cigarettes, but they are not good for you either!

Douching for odor and/or increased discharge is like a dog chasing it's own tail since it causes BV and Yeast infections that produce both symptoms by washing away the good organisms that keep the bad ones in check. While douching may temporarily relieve your symptoms, it does not get at the root of your problem, the infection itself. The infection continues to produce the odor and/or increased discharge that makes you douche over and over again!

Douching causes more serious pelvic infections involving your uterus, tubes and ovaries, particularly if you do it after your period. During your period the opening to your uterus is wider than usual to let your blood flow out. Your blood is good food for the smaller amounts of bacteria that are normally present so their numbers subsequently increase. Douching after your period flushes this nasty bacterial soup up inside your uterus.

14

Desqumative Inflammatory Vaginitis

Desquamative Inflammatory Vaginitis—also called "DIV"—is also in the bacterial class of germ organisms.

Although DIV is also an overgrowth of bacteria, it differs from BV since it irritates your vagina, causes its walls to peel, any type of bacteria can overgrow-aerobic as well as anaerobic-with each woman having her own unique set of overgrown bacteria.

SYMPTOMS

DIV causes a yellow frothy vaginal discharge that frequently has an odor.

DIV also causes itching, burning, redness and/or swelling of your vulva and vagina that frequently causes pain during sex.

Again, none of these symptoms are unique to DIV since they also occur with other infections and conditions or infections. For instance, itching and burning is also common when you have Yeast and/or Trichomonas, which also causes a yellow frothy discharge.

DIAGNOSIS

Since DIV is not well understood, it is EXTREMELY HARD TO DIAGNOSE. Most gynecologists are not even aware of it so do not be surprised if it is missed. I was only made aware of it 4 years ago by an Infectious Disease specialist after seeking his advice for additional treatments for what I mistakenly thought was an extremely resistant strain of Trichomonas.

Generally, it is diagnosed only after you have not responded to Metronidazole for a presumed Trichomonas infection.

Again, you should SPECIFICALLY REQUEST A SALINE PREP if you have itching and/or a lot of discharge, especially if your vulva, vagina and/or cervix appear irritated. Generally, it reveals lots of inflammatory white cells and bacteria without the clue cells that are seen in BV. This saline prep is discussed in detail in the Yeast chapter and, again, it is difficult to interpret your saline prep during your period, after you douche, if you have more than one infection or after mistakenly inserting an over-the-counter (OTC) Yeast medication.

Again, at times a drop of potassium hydroxide is added for a KOH WHIFF test. If there is no fishy odor, you most likely have DIV and not BV.

Again, your saline prep is more accurate when it is performed regularly by your medical professional rather than once in a while since practice makes perfect.

Again, beware of medical professionals who rely on the appearance of your discharge and/or your PAP smear result alone! I cannot tell you how many times I was fooled into thinking that Yeast always looked like cottage cheese or that Trichomonas always had to be frothy yellow only to be proved wrong under the microscope. The PAP was designed for pre-cancerous and cancerous cervical changes, not infection so it misses far more of them than it ever picks up! It also takes 5 to 14 days for your results to come back.

Again, although bacteria are sometimes MENTIONED ON YOUR PAP report, this does not mean that you actually have an infection because they are normally found on your vagina and cervix.

Again, CULTURING IS OF NO USE since bacteria are always present in your vagina.

Again, we often test you for Gonorrhea and Chlamydia (see both of these chapters) because they also cause a lot of discharge and/or an irritated cervix and are not seen easily under the microscope.

TREATMENT

We also treat DIV with Clindamycin /Cleocin-2% antibiotic vaginal cream and/or suppository-ovules at bedtime, but for 6 to 7 days instead of the usual 3-night BV course. Unfortunately, there is a 30% relapse rate and you may need a second week. It also comes in oral or mouth tablets, but the cream works better since it is directly applied to the irritated surfaces. If you get your period, try to resume it afterwards.

Again, you should consider using a one-night OTC anti-fungal since antibiotics might cause an overgrowth of Yeast.

Prescription Sultrin cream, OTC anti-fungals and anti-itch preparations like A+D, Vagisil, Vaginex, Vagicaine, Benzocaine, Lanicaine, Cortizone, Cortaid, Gynecort and Summer's Eve Medicated WILL NOT TREAT DIV, only make it worse!

DOUCHING

For the fourth time, I feel compelled to review the Douching Section.

Douching, feminine deodorants and powders never clean you so they are not recommended for routine hygiene, odor or increased discharge!

Douching only puts money in the pockets of men who do not! Do not assume that being able to purchase them makes them good for you, as the deceptive advertising would have you believe. You can also buy alcohol and cigarettes, but they aren't good for you either!

Douching for odor and/or increased discharge is like a dog chasing it's own tail since it causes BV and Yeast infections that produce both symptoms by washing away the good organisms that keep the bad ones in check. While douching may temporarily relieve your symptoms, it does not get at the root of your problem, the infection itself. The infection continues to produce the odor and/or increased discharge that makes you douche over and over again!

Douching causes more serious pelvic infections involving your uterus, tubes and ovaries, particularly if you do it after your period. During your period the opening to your uterus is wider than usual to let your blood flow out. Your blood is good food for the smaller amounts of bacteria that are normally present so their numbers subsequently increase. Douching after your period flushes this nasty bacterial soup up inside your uterus.

15

Gonorrhea

Gonorrhea—also called "GC", "the clap" or "the drip"—infects 600,000 Americans each year. It is included in the bacteria class of germ organisms.

TRANSMISSION

GC is a STD or SEXUALLY TRANSMITTED DISEASE that is passed from person-to-person through close intimate sexual contact, including acts other than vaginal-penile penetration. This includes those of you who have female-to-female sex and even you so-called virgins who engage in "heavy petting" without actually being penetrated!

TRANSLATION: He doesn't have to stick it in for you to get it! Just having his penis in the vicinity of the outside vulva and vaginal orifice is enough for you to get it!

You can also pass it on to your newborn's eyes during birth and this is why they are given antibiotic eye drops soon afterwards!

You cannot get GC from soiled towels, underwear, and/or bathing suits nor from a moist toilet seat, steam room, sauna, jacuzzi, chlorinated pool or hot tub!

INFECTION SITES

GC can infect any or all of the sites listed below.

Cervix	Urethra	Throat
Uterus	Skene's glands	Eyes
Tubes	Bartholin's glands	Liver surface
Ovaries	Rectum	Ankle, knee and wrist joints

COMPLICATIONS

GC can travel from your cervix up into your uterus, tubes and ovaries along with other bacteria living in your vagina to cause a serious pelvic infection. This is commonly referred to as or "Salpingitis" or "PID" and they are both discussed in their own chapter.

Salpingitis-PID causes scar tissue to form and this results in:

1. **Sterility** or inability to get pregnant since 20% have a complete blockage of their tubes.
2. Life-threatening **tubal pregnancies** if your tubes are partially blocked.
3. **Chronic pelvic pain**, especially when you have sex, in 15 to 20%.

GC infection during pregnancy also causes:

1. **Miscarriage.**
2. **Premature labor.**
3. **Premature membrane rupture.**
4. **Premature delivery** with the possibility of a newborn eye infection.
5. **Uterine infections** that may complicate your miscarriage, abortion, vaginal delivery or Cesarean section.

SYMPTOMS

You can have NO SYMPTOMS or any of the following.

1. **An increase in your usual discharge or a yellow one.**
2. Dull achy, persistent **pain in your lower abdomen** above your mons hairline.
3. **Pain during sex** that usually interrupts it.
4. **Pain when you urinate** that possibly makes feel like you can't hold it, makes your urinate a lot or urinate little bits at a time.
5. Painful mass on either side of your vaginal entrance.
6. Fever.
7. Rectal pain.
8. Pain during unsuccessful attempts to have a bowel movement, which passes only blood and mucus produced instead.
9. Sore throat with persistent cough.
10. One or two painful, red, swollen wrist, finger, knee or ankle joints with an overlying skin rash.
11. Pain in the right upper portion of your abdomen.

DIAGNOSIS

In women, GC TESTING IS ROUTINE since it can damage your tubes!

The DNA-PROBE is the most popular test since the results only take 24 hours and Chlamydia can be tested for simultaneously. This is a similar bacterial STD, which infects 4 million Americans a year and is present in 20% to 40% of those with Gonorrhea. Your cervix is swabbed with a regular-sized Q-tip as long as you are not bleeding OR your urethra with a thinner metal one. Either Q-tip is then placed in a special plastic tube with a special solution. Occasionally, you are given a special plastic cup to take home in order to collect the first urine of the day.

GC can also be CULTURED after Q-tip swabbing of your cervix whether you are bleeding or not, urethra, throat, anus, eye and/or Bartholin's gland or after joint fluid is obtained after inserting a needle under local anesthesia. The Q-tip or joint fluid is smeared onto a special refrigerated plate with sheep blood gelatin. Then we keep it warm in a special oxygen-poor environment until it is ready to be analyzed 48 hours later. It is cheaper, but less convenient.

A positive GC result is usually reported to the health departments of many cities and counties.

A lot of you look at me like I am stark raving mad when I tell you that you have a STD, yet you have not had sex for a while. I hate to burst your bubble, but mad I am not.

STD'S DO NOT GO AWAY JUST BECAUSE YOU STOP HAVING SEX!

You get STD's from sex, but the opposite is not true. An STD like Gonorrhea is more than happy to live inside you until you die—with or without sex—since your body supplies everything it needs to survive!

TREATMENT

We treat uncomplicated GC infections of your cervix, urethra, Bartholin's glands, rectum and throat with any of the ONE-DOSE antibiotics below.

1. **Cefixime** / Suprax 400mg by mouth (which is generally used in pregnancy).
2. **Ofloxacin** / Floxin 400mg again by mouth.
3. **Ciprofloxacin** / Cipro 500mg also by mouth.
4. **Ceftriazone** / Rocephin 125mg injected into one buttock.

More complicated joint infections require hospitalization for one of the intravenous antibiotics above.

DOUCHING

For the fifth time, I feel compelled to review the Douching Section, but with a new twist!

Douching can give you salpingitis-PID by flushing GC up inside your uterus and tubes from your cervix where it was originally.

Douching can give you salpingitis-PID even if you do not have GC, particularly if you do it after your period. During your period the opening to your uterus is wider than usual to let your blood flow out. Your blood is good food for the smaller amounts of bacteria that are normally present so their numbers subsequently increase. Douching after your period flushes this nasty bacterial soup up inside your uterus.

Douching, feminine deodorants and powders never clean you so they are not recommended for routine hygiene, odor or increased discharge!

Douching only puts money in the pockets of men who do not! Do not assume that being able to purchase them makes them good for you, as the deceptive advertising would have you believe. You can also buy alcohol and cigarettes, but they aren't good for you either!

Douching for odor and/or increased discharge is like a dog chasing it's own tail since it causes BV and Yeast infections that produce both symptoms by washing away your good organisms that keep your bad ones in check. While douching may temporarily relieve your symptoms, it does not get at the root of your problem, the infection itself. The infection continues to produce the odor and/or increased discharge that makes you douche over and over again!

MALE INFECTION

Again, since GC is a STD it would be criminal not to arm you with information about this infection in men!

Again, it primarily INFECTS their much longer penile urethra. Rarely, it infects their prostate and epididymis, which are both defined in the Trichomonas Chapter.

Usually they have no symptoms or urinary ones if present. Sometimes there is pain at the bottom of their bladder and/or their SCROTUM or the wrinkled skin sac encasing the epididymis and TESTICLES or balls.

GC is detected by the same methods routinely used with women, but only men with symptoms and/or suspicious discharge tend to be tested. Apparently, it is too uncomfortable for the entire penile urethra to be sampled with the thin metal Q-tip swab. Obviously, it is still a Man's World since undressing and having a speculum in your vagina is probably just as uncomfortable!

Usually their urine and/or discharge are microscopically examined instead for inflammatory white cells that have GC organisms trapped inside of them. Again, an Urologist is the best medical professional to do this since practice makes perfect.

Your male partner needs to specifically say, "My partner has Gonorrhea" as opposed to vague stuff like "My girl said I gave her an infection." This only sends the medical professional on a wild goose chase and more often than not results in a missed diagnosis since there are many types of infections. There is no need for the medical professional to be tortured with a game of "Twenty Questions" when they are simply trying to help!

TREATMENT is similar for uncomplicated urethral and rectal infections. Complicated prostatitis, epididymitis require a 2-week course of Floxin or Cipro. Again, IV antibiotics are used for joint infections.

Your partner should be treated 48 hours or more before you resume sex or your treatment will be wasted!

Do not be surprised if you are a double-dose of medication to share with your partner, though you should encourage him or her to seek separate testing and treatment. Make sure you question your partner about medication allergies before you treat him or her.

Again, being treated once will not prevent you from getting GC again from the same or different partner! Once again, barrier protection will lower your chances of infection.

16

Chlamydia and LGV

Chlamydia infects 4 million Americans each year. It is included in the bacteria class of germ organisms, although it has some features of a virus as well as a parasite. Specifically speaking, it is an "intracellular obligate parasite" and its mixed features delayed its discovery until the 1940's.

TRANSMISSION

Chlamydia is a STD or SEXUALLY-TRANSMITTED DISEASE that is passed from person-to-person through close intimate sexual contact, including acts other than vaginal-penile penetration. This includes female-to-female sex and so-called virgins who engage in "heavy petting" without actually being penetrated!

TRANSLATION: He doesn't have to stick it in for you to get it! Just having his penis in the vicinity of the outside vulva and vaginal orifice is enough for you to get it!

You can also pass it on to your newborn's eyes during birth and this is why they are given antibiotic eye drops soon afterwards! It can even infect their lings and, rarely, their ears.

You cannot get Chlamydia from soiled towels, underwear, and/or bathing suits nor from a moist toilet seat, steam room, sauna, jacuzzi, chlorinated pool or hot tub!

INFECTION SITES

Chlamydia infects any or all of the sites below.

Cervix	Urethra	Eyes
Uterus	Skene's glands	Throats
Tubes	Bartholin's glands	Liver surface
Ovaries	Rectum	Joints

COMPLICATIONS

Chlamydia can travel from your cervix up into your uterus, tubes and ovaries along with other bacteria living in your vagina to cause a serious pelvic infection. This is commonly referred to as or "Salpingitis" or "PID" and they are both discussed in their own chapter.

Salpingitis-PID causes scar tissue to form and this results in:

1. **Sterility** or inability to get pregnant since 20% have a complete blockage of their tubes.
2. Life-threatening **tubal pregnancies** if your tubes are partially blocked.
3. **Chronic pelvic pain**, especially when you have sex, in 15 to 20%.

GC infection during pregnancy also causes:

1. **Miscarriage.**
2. **Premature labor.**
3. **Premature membrane rupture.**
4. **Premature delivery** with the possibility of a newborn eye infection.
5. **Uterine infections** that may complicate your miscarriage, abortion, vaginal delivery or Cesarean section.

SYMPTOMS

You can have NO SYMPTOMS or any of the following.

1. **An increase in your usual discharge or a yellow one.**
2. Dull achy, persistent **pain in your lower abdomen** above your mons hairline.
3. **Pain during sex** that usually interrupts it.
4. **Pain when you urinate** that possibly makes feel like you can't hold it, makes your urinate a lot or urinate little bits at a time.
5. Painful mass on either side of your vaginal entrance.
6. Fever.
7. Rectal pain.
8. Pain during unsuccessful attempts to have a bowel movement, which passes only blood and mucus produced instead.
9. Sore throat with persistent cough.
10. One or two painful, red, swollen wrist, finger, knee or ankle joints with an overlying skin rash.
11. Pain in the right upper portion of your abdomen.
12. Reiter's Syndrome consisting of red runny eyes in association with swollen painful joints and skin rash.

DIAGNOSIS

In women, CHLAMYDIA TESTING IS ROUTINE since it can damage your tubes!

The DNA-PROBE is the most popular test since the results only take 24 hours and Gonorrhea can be tested for simultaneously. This is a similar bacterial STD, which infects 600,000 Americans a year and is present in 20% to 40% of those with Chlamydia. Your cervix is swabbed with a regular-sized Q-tip as long as you are not bleeding OR your urethra with a thinner metal one. Either Q-tip is then placed in a special plastic tube with a special solution. Occasionally, you are given a special plastic cup to take home in order to collect the first urine of the day.

Chlamydia can also be CULTURED in a special Chlamydia or viral solution from a Q-tip that was swabbed inside your cervix whether you are bleeding or not, urethra, throat or rectum. This is more expensive, takes 7 to 10 days and must be kept refrigerated before and after or Chlamydia will die.

OTHER less accurate methods include antigen tests that detect a portion of the Chlamydia organism, antibody tests that detect substances that your body makes in response to Chlamydia and enzyme tests that detect substances that Chlamydia needs to survive.

A positive Chlamydia test result is usually reported to the health departments of many cities and counties.

A lot of you look at me like I am stark raving mad when I tell you that you have a STD, yet you have not had sex for a while. I hate to burst your bubble, but mad I am not.

STD'S DO NOT GO AWAY JUST BECAUSE YOU STOP HAVING SEX!

You get STD's from sex, but the opposite is not true. An STD like Chlamydia is more than happy to live inside you until you die—with or without sex—since your body supplies everything it needs to survive!

TREATMENT

We treat uncomplicated Chlamydial infections of your cervix, urethra, Bartholin's glands, rectum and throat with any of the antibiotics below.

1. **Azithromycin** / Zithromax 1 gram in a single dose which is convenient, but expensive.
2. **Ofloxacin** / Floxin 300mg twice daily for 7 days which is the most expensive.
3. **Doxycycline** / Vibramycin or Doryx 100 mg twice daily for 7 days which is cheapest, but you should avoid it if you are pregnant.
4. **Erythromycin** 500mg four times daily for 7 days which is also cheap, but it upsets your stomach so much that you probably won't finish it!

More complicated Reiter's Syndrome requires a longer 2-week course of Floxin, Doxycycline and/or Erythromycin.

DOUCHING

For the sixth time, I feel compelled to review the Douching Section, again with a new twist!

Douching can give you salpingitis-PID by flushing Chlamydia up inside your uterus and tubes from your cervix where it was originally.

Douching can give you salpingitis-PID even if you do not have Chlamydia, particularly if you do it after your period. During your period the opening to your uterus is wider than usual to let your blood flow out. Your blood is good food for the smaller amounts of bacteria that are normally present so their numbers subsequently increase. Douching after your period flushes this nasty bacterial soup up inside your uterus.

Douching, feminine deodorants and powders never clean you so they are not recommended for routine hygiene, odor or increased discharge!

Douching only puts money in the pockets of men who do not! Do not assume that being able to purchase them makes them good for you, as the deceptive advertising would have you believe. You can also buy alcohol and cigarettes, but they aren't good for you either!

Douching for odor and/or increased discharge is like a dog chasing it's own tail since it causes BV and Yeast infections that produce both symptoms by washing away your good organisms that keep your bad ones in check. While douching may temporarily relieve your symptoms, it does not get at the root of your problem, the infection itself. The infection continues to produce the odor and/or increased discharge that makes you douche over and over again!

MALE INFECTION

Again, since Chlamydia is a STD it would be criminal not to arm you with information about this infection in men!

Again, it primarily INFECTS their much longer penile urethra. Rarely, it infects their prostate and epididymis, which are both defined in the Trichomonas Chapter.

Usually, they have NO SYMPTOMS or urinary ones if present. Sometimes they report pain at the bottom of the bladder and/or inside the SCROTUM or the wrinkled skin sac encasing the epididymis and TESTICLES or balls.

Chlamydia is detected by the same methods routinely used with women, but only men with symptoms and/or suspicious discharge

tend to be tested. Apparently, it is too uncomfortable for their entire penile urethra to be sampled with the thin metal Q-tip swab. Obviously, it is still a Man's World since undressing and having a speculum in your vagina is probably just as uncomfortable!

Usually, urine or penile discharge is examined under the microscope for Non-Gonococcal Urethritis (NGU) or inflammatory white cells that do not have GC organisms trapped inside of them. Again, Urologists are the best medical professionals to do this test since practice makes perfect. Even so, only 23 to 55% actually have Chlamydia since other infections and conditions cause the same findings!

USUALLY THERE IS NO TESTING FOR AT ALL and treatment prescribed solely for a having a sexual partner with Chlamydia!

Your male partner needs to specifically say, "My partner has Chlamydia" as opposed to vague stuff like "My girl said I gave her an infection." This only sends the medical professional on a wild goose chase and more often than not results in a missed diagnosis since there are many types of infections. There is no need for the medical professional to be tortured with a game of "Twenty Questions" when they are simply trying to help!

TREATMENT is similar for uncomplicated urethral, rectal and throat infections, with generally 2-week courses of Floxin or Doxycycline required for epididymitis and Reiter's Syndrome.

Your partner should be treated 48 hours or more before you resume sex or your treatment will be wasted!

Do not be surprised if you are given a double-dose of medication to share with your partner, though you should encourage him or her to seek separate testing and treatment. Make sure you question your partner about medication allergies before giving it, however.

Again, being treated once will not prevent you from getting Chlamydia again from the same or different partner! Once again, barrier protection will lower your chances of infection.

LGV

LGV or Lympho-Granuloma Venereum results from extremely rare and particularly aggressive strains of Chlamydia that invade your vulva, vagina and cervix.

Initially, there is a painful dime to quarter sized sore at the entry site, which eventually heals over in a few weeks, though sometimes you never see it.

Next, a BULBO or painful abcessed lymph node forms in your INGUINAL or thigh-hip skin fold that is typically the size of a peanut shell or larger as Chlamydia travels through and destroys the lymph channels that normally drain infection.

Generally, we rely on blood testing for Chlamydia antibodies to confirm it since so much time has passed from your initial infection before it is recognized

Treatment consists of 3-to 6-week courses of Zithromax once a week or daily Doxycycline and Erythromycin as well as surgical drainage if indicated.

Again, LGV is usually reported to most health departments and do not be surprised if they actually contact you since it is so rare.

17

Salpingitis—PID

Salpingitis is a continuous pelvic infection from your cervix to your uterus to your tubes and to your ovaries, even though "salpinges" means "tubes" in Latin. The infecting germ organisms are bacteria.

COMPLICATIONS

Salpingitis causes scar tissue to form and this results in:

1. **Sterility** or inability to get pregnant since 20% have a complete blockage of their tubes.
2. Life-threatening **tubal pregnancies** if your tubes are partially blocked.
3. **Chronic pelvic pain**, especially when you have sex, in 15 to 20%.

PELVIC INFLAMMATORY DISEASE

A lot of medical professionals incorrectly use the term "Pelvic Inflammatory Disease" or "PID" for salpingitis. This is a poor substitute however, since all of the pelvic conditions below inflame or irritate your pelvis.

1. Bladder infections (see UTI Chapter).
2. Appendicitis.
3. Symptomatic uterine fibroid tumors (see this chapter).
4. Symptomatic ovarian cysts (see this chapter).
5. Symptomatic adhesions or scar tissue.
6. Endometriosis (see this chapter).
7. Food and/or water-borne infectious diarrhea.
8. Inflammatory bowel disease.
9. Irritable bowel syndrome.
10. Cancers of the ovaries, tubes, uterus, cervix, rectum and bladder.

CAUSES

Salpingitis starts as a Gonorrhea (GC) and/or Chlamydia cervical infection(s) in 90% of cases. They are both STD's or SEXUALLY-TRANSMITTED DISEASES that are passed from person-to-person through close intimate sexual contact, including acts other than vaginal-penile penetration. GC is also seen in 20 to 40% of the 4 million Americans with Chlamydia and Chlamydia is seen in 20 to 40% of the 600,000 Americans with GC.

The remaining 10% of cases occur after DOUCHING, miscarriage, abortion, vaginal delivery, Cesarean section, other pelvic surgeries or after HIV infection leads to AIDS.

DOUCHING

Here we go again, but for the last time! Of course, salpingitis is the most important reason not to douche!

Douching can give you salpingitis-PID by flushing GC and Chlamydia up inside your uterus and tubes from your cervix where it was originally.

Douching can give you salpingitis-PID even if you do not have these STD's, particularly if you do it after your period. During your period the opening to your uterus is wider than usual to let your blood flow out. Your blood is good food for the smaller amounts of bacteria that are normally present so their numbers subsequently increase. Douching after your period flushes this nasty bacterial soup up inside your uterus.

Douching, feminine deodorants and powders never clean you so they are not recommended for routine hygiene, odor or increased discharge!

Douching only puts money in the pockets of men who do not! Do not assume that being able to purchase them makes them good for you, as the deceptive advertising would have you believe. You can also buy alcohol and cigarettes, but they aren't good for you either!

Douching for odor and/or increased discharge is like a dog chasing it's own tail since it causes BV and Yeast infections that produce both symptoms by washing away your good organisms that keep your bad ones in check. While douching may temporarily relieve your symptoms, it does not get at the root of your problem, the infection itself. The infection continues to produce the odor and/or increased discharge that makes you douche over and over again!

SYMPTOMS

Typically, you have any of the SYMPTOMS below.

1. **An increase in your usual discharge or a yellow one** and possibly odor as well.
2. **Dull achy, persistent pain in your lower abdomen** above your mons hairline.

3. **Pain during sex that** usually interrupts it.
4. Fever.
5. Fatigue.

You could even have symptoms related to GC and/or Chlamydia elsewhere.

1. Pain when you urinate that possibly makes feel like you can't hold it, makes your urinate a lot or urinate little bits at a time.
2. Painful mass on either side of your vaginal entrance.
3. Rectal pain.
4. Pain during unsuccessful attempts to have a bowel movement, which passes only blood and mucus produced instead.
5. Sore throat with persistent cough.
6. One or two painful, red, swollen wrist, finger, knee or ankle joints with an overlying skin rash.
7. Pain in the right upper portion of your abdomen.

DIAGNOSIS

YOUR PHYSICAL EXAM *MUST* SHOW:

1. **A lot of discharge and an inflamed red cervix** upon speculum inspection (see the Pelvic Exam Chapter).
2. **Significant tenderness of your cervix, uterus and adnexa** during your bimanual Exam.
3. **No rectal mass, diarrhea or blood in your stool** during your rectovaginal exam since this usually indicates a separate GI or Gastro-Intestinal problem.

YOUR PHYSICAL EXAM *MIGHT* ALSO SHOW:

1. **An enlarged mass on one or both sides of your uterus** during your bimanual exam that could be an adnexal abcess or pus pocket if your infection is severe.

2. **Significant tenderness of your lower abdomen** when we press down lightly.

ADDITIONAL TESTS ARE ALSO SENT INCLUDING:

1. **Mandatory pregnancy testing** since tubal pregnancy causes similar pain symptoms.
2. **Mandatory GC and Chlamydia testing from your cervix.**
3. **Urine culturing** to exclude a bacterial bladder infection (see UTI Chapter) that causes similar pain symptoms as well.
4. **Stool testing for bacterial culture and parasites** if you have diarrhea.
5. **Blood testing to check your liver, gallbladder and pancreas** if you have nausea, vomiting, poor appetite and right upper quadrant abdominal pain since this could indicate a separate GI problem (though rarely GC and Chlamydia infects your surface).
6. **Blood testing to see if the white cells that help you fight infection are high.**
7. **Blood testing for check for Syphilis** since this is another STD and STD's tend to travel together!
8. **Pelvic sonogram** if you are too tender to tolerate a complete pelvic exam or an abcess is suspected.
9. **Laparoscopy surgery under anesthesia** that introduces a telescope through a small incision under your belly button if we suspect a tubal pregnancy or if your diagnosis is unclear.

Many cases of salpingitis-PID are never diagnosed, particularly if your symptoms are mild. Unfortunately you can still have a lot of tubal damage even if your symptoms are mild since your infection can go untreated for a long time.

We estimate that there are 1,000,000 cases of salpingitis-PID each year in the US. Unfortunately, this figure is not very accurate because many inexperienced medical professionals over-diagnose salpingitis-PID when another form of PID is present.

This tendency to over-diagnose is tolerated because of the tubal damage that often results without treatment. Keep this in mind when you get a preliminary diagnosis of "PID" from an Emergency Room, Clinic or Office Visit. Make sure you call back for the results of any GC, Chlamydia and/or urine culture tests that might confirm or exclude actual salpingitis-PID. Be sure to go back if your symptoms persist despite treatment because you may need further tests to determine your correct diagnosis. Even expert gynecologists were wrong 25% of the time in a study where laparoscopy was used to see if their suspected salpingitis-PID diagnosis was indeed correct.

TREATMENT

SALPINGITIS-PID ORAL ANTIBIOTIC TREATMENT lasts for 7 to 14 days and has to cover GC, Chlamydia and all of the other bacteria involved.

1. Metronidazole / Flagyl 500mg along with Ofloxacin / Floxin 400mg both twice daily which is the simplest, though expensive.
2. Amoxacillin-Clavulanic acid / Augmentin 500mg thrice daily with meals, Doxycycline 100mg twice daily for Chlamydia and one of 3 possible single-dose GC therapies namely, Floxin 400mg or Ciprofloxacin / Cipro 500mg or Cefixime / Suprax 400mg.
3. Flagyl 500mg and Doxycycline 100mg both twice daily along with one of the single-dose GC therapies above which is the cheapest, yet least effective.
4. Flagyl 500 mg twice daily and Amoxacillin 500mg thrice daily along with single-dose Azithromycin / Zithromax 1 gram for Chlamydia and one of the single-dose GC therapies above which is complicated and expensive.

Never douching again, no sex and/or tampons for 4 to 6 weeks, bedrest, good nutrition, ample fluids, non-narcotic pain medications are all suggested as well as anti-vomiting and anti-diarrhea when indicated.

You may even become one of the 200,000 to 300,000 women in the US each year WHO REQUIRE HOSPITALIZATION FOR STRONGER IV ANTIBIOTICS IF:

1. **There is no improvement after 2 to 3 days** of oral antibiotics!
2. **You are an adolescent or do not have any children** to limit the damage to your tubes and preserve your fertility.
3. **Vomiting is so severe** that your oral antibiotics won't stay down.
4. **There is a fever greater than 100.4F.**
5. **The pain is so severe that narcotic pain injections are required.**
6. **An abcess** is suspected on your bimanual exam and/or sonogram.
7. **An IUD is present that should also be removed as soon as possible** since it makes this infection worse.
8. **A pregnancy is present** since miscarriage could result and also make this infection worse.
9. **HIV, especially if it has progressed to AIDS.**
10. **The diagnosis is uncertain.**

IF YOU DO NOT RESPOND TO IV ANTIBIOTICS, PELVIC SURGERY may be needed to drain your abcess(es) and probably remove your diseased uterus, tubes, ovaries and cervix as well.

Your partner should also be treated for GC and Chlamydia! Again, do not be surprised if your partner tells you no testing was done since most medical professionals that they see will simply write out a prescription, especially if they do not have symptoms. Being treated once for GC and Chlamydia will not keep you from getting it again from the same or different partner though barrier protection will lower your chances of re-infection.

18

Urinary Tract Infection

Urinary Tract Infection—called "UTI" for short—is an infection of the urinary tract, which consists of your urethra, bladder and URETERS or tubes that run from each side of your bladder to each kidney.

The lower tract consists of your urethra and bladder and the upper tract consists of your kidneys and the ureters. UTI's usually begin at your urethra and travel up to your bladder, ureters and kidneys, though sometimes they begin in your kidney and travel on down if you have stones.

The appropriate medical terms for these infections are:

1. URETHRITIS if only your urethra is infected.
2. CYSTITIS if your bladder and urethra are both infected.
3. PYELONEPHRITIS if your kidney, ureter, bladder and urethra are all infected.

SYMPTOMS

LOWER TRACT infections may or may not cause:

1. **DYSURIA** or pain when you urinate and this can be virtually teeth clenching as I found out!
2. **Frequency** or urinating a lot.
3. **Urgency** or feeling like you cannot hold it.
4. **Dribbling** or urinating a little bit at a time.
5. **HEMATURIA** or blood in your urine.
6. **Pain over your mons** area.
7. Low-grade fever that is generally **less than 100.3 F.**

UPPER TRACT infections generally cause any of those above as well as fever over 100.4F and/or RENAL COLIC, which is back pain that starts below your bottom rib where each kidney is located then curves around the side of your lower abdomen along the course of each ureter towards your bladder in front.

URETHRITIS ORGANISMS

Yeast fungus along with STD's like Trichomonas parasite, Gonorrhea (GC) and/or Chlamydia bacteria, Herpes and/or Wart virus all infect your urethra and are all mentioned in their own separate chapters.

STD's or SEXUALLY-TRANSMITTED DISEASES are passed from person-to-person through close intimate sexual contact, including acts other than vaginal-penile penetration. This includes those of you who have female-to-female sex and even you so-called virgins who engage in "heavy petting" without actually being penetrated!

TRANSLATION: He doesn't have to stick it in for you to get a disease! Just having his penis in the vicinity of the outside vulva and vaginal orifice is enough for you to get a disease!

On the other hand, Yeast fungus normally lives in small numbers all over your body as well as inside many of its cavities. A Yeast infection results when it grows too much.

URETHRITIS DIAGNOSIS

Urethritis is usually diagnosed when your urethral meatus is red and irritated with a milky or yellow discharge on visual inspection instead of a being pink with the usual clear mucus.

A thin Q-tip is briefly twirled inside your urethra for simultaneous DNA probe GC and Chlamydia testing or separate GC and Chlamydia culturing in special growth solutions since they will not grow in a regular bacterial culture.

If tiny blister-type sores are seen they are presumed to be herpes, though this can be confirmed by also swabbing them with a Q-tip, which is then placed in a special viral solution before being transported to an outside lab.

If cauliflower growths are seen they are presumed to be warts, especially if you have more of them elsewhere. Generally, they do not cause any other symptoms and further testing is rarely except for the occasional biopsy if they do not have this characteristic appearance.

If your vaginal orifice is also red and irritated you also need a speculum exam to possibly swab your cervix for GC and Chlamydia again and to obtain discharge for a microscopic Saline Prep test (see the Yeast Chapter) to check for yeast forms, moving and/or nonmonving Trichomonads organisms, inflammatory white cells, clue cells and bacteria.

A clean-catch/mid-stream urine should have been given before your exam by first wiping yourself clean from your urethral meatus to your vaginal orifice. Then you flip the toilet seat up, straddle the toilet without sitting on it and urinate while passing a sterile container only under the middle portion of one continuous urine stream without starting and stopping.

A specially prepared stick is dipped into one portion of the urine in the office to test for inflammatory white cells and red blood cells.

If might also be examined under a microscope in the office or an outside lab outside to look for bacteria, swimming Trichomonad organisms and yeast forms as well as the inflammatory white cells and red blood cells again.

The rest of your urine might be sent to an outside lab to be cultured for bacteria over the next 24 to 48 hours. If the result shows no growth, urethritis is confirmed.

A lot of you look at me like I am stark raving mad when I tell you that you have a STD, yet you have not had sex for a while. I hate to burst your bubble, but mad I am not.

STD'S DO NOT GO AWAY JUST BECAUSE YOU STOP HAVING SEX!

You get STD's from sex, but the opposite is not true. STD's are more than happy to live inside you until you die—with or without sex—since your body supplies everything they need to survive!

URETHRITIS TREATMENT

Urethritis treatment depends on the organism you are infected with.

1. **Yeast** responds to several over-the-counter (OTC) and prescription anti-fungals.
2. **Trichomonas** is cured by Metronidazole / Flagyl.
3. **GC** requires a single-dose of Suprax, Floxin and Cipro.
4. **Chlamydia** requires a week of Floxin, Cipro, Doxycycline and Erythromycin or single-dose Zithromax.

5. **Herpes** responds to Zovirax, Valterx and Famvir if it is severe cases or simply time if it is not.
6. **Warts** can be destroyed by freezing or applying 10 to 15% Podophyllin Compound weekly both in the office.

CYSTITIS

Cystitis is diagnosed when one bacteria grows significantly in your urine culture. If two or more bacteria grow in your urine culture you did not give it correctly and contaminating vaginal discharge, blood and/or skin that also have bacteria was mixed in with your urine.

We treat cystitis oral antibiotics that are usually given for 2 to 7 days. We start them without the culture results if you have symptoms and sometimes the antibiotic is switched if it does not kill the bacteria that subsequently grew out on your culture1 to 2 days later.

Unfortunately many medical professionals incorrectly assume cystitis is the only type of UTI possible whenever you report lower tract urinary symptoms and have inflammatory white cells and/or red blood cells on your office urine dipstick. Most will not even examine you!

Trichomoniacal urethritis, Yeast urethritis, GC urethritis, Chlamydial urethritis, Herpes urethritis and cystitis all cause the same symptoms and dipstick findings. Cystitis treatment does little or nothing for the others, however!

PYELONEPHRITIS

Pyelonephritis is diagnosed when you have fever, back pain, possibly lower tract symptoms and significant bacterial growth in your urine culture.

Generally you need to be hospitalized for intravenous antibiotics for a few days since it is easy for bacteria to spread to your bloodstream given the extremely dense composition of your kidneys and the large amount of blood that is filtered through them.

Then we send you home on a longer 10 to 14-day course of oral antibiotics.

A kidney stone should also be suspected, if there is a lot of blood in your urine. To confirm this, you may have to strain your urine while additional tests are performed.

OTHER TREATMENTS

Prescription Phenozopyridine / Pyridium and OTC Uristat are urinary tract anesthetics that relieve your urinary symptoms since it takes 6 to 12 hoursyou're your antibiotic to kick in. It makes your urine bright orange, but you'll definitely appreciate it!

Cranberry juice and OTC Azo both contain Hippuric acid, a natural antibiotic.

Try to urinate right after sex to flush bacteria away from your urethra that might have been carried there by your partner's penis, mouth or fingers.

Use barrier protection to lower your chance of getting a STD, though keep in mind that male condoms do nothing for herpes and warts that are not on or inside his penis!

19

Genital Herpes

Genital herpes is included in the viral class of germ organisms since they are caused by an infection with Herpes Simplex Virus or HSV.

Over 45 million Americans have some form of herpes—myself included—though most are not aware of it!

INFECTION SITES

Herpes can infect any or all of the sites below.

Oral lips and mouth	Bladder	Nose
Vulva	Perineum	Nail cuticles
Vagina	Anus and Rectum	Liver
Cervix	Buttocks crease	Nerves to all of these areas
Urethra	Eyes	Brain itself

TRANSMISSION

Herpes is a STD or SEXUALLY-TRANSMITTED DISEASE that is passed from person-to-person through close intimate sexual contact, including acts other than vaginal-penile penetration. This includes female-to-female sex as well as so-called virgins who engage in "heavy petting" without actually being penetrated!

TRANSLATION: He doesn't have to stick it in for you to get it! Just having his penis in the vicinity of your vulva and vaginal orifice is enough for you to get it!

It is important to remember that male condoms will not protect you from warts that are not on or inside his penis.

You can also pass it to your newborn during pregnancy and childbirth, though generally this involves a first-time genital infection during the 7th to 9th month that frequently leads to premature labor and/or membrane rupture. If you deliver at this time, you have not yet made any protective anti-herpes antibodies to transfer to your newborn since it takes 6 to 12 weeks to make them. As a result of this, newborn herpes is particularly with death occurring in 50% and significant brain damage in another 25%!

Cold sores or fever blisters are also herpes, but it was not passed to you during sex, for the most part. You can spread herpes from this area to your genitals, eyes or nose if you pick at a fresh cold sore then touch these areas without washing your hands first.

In rare cases you can get it from a warm soiled towel, underwear or bathing suit that has just been used by someone else, but if you do this you are probable having sex with that person. You can't get herpes from soiled towels, underwear or bathing suits that have been sitting around for a while, a moist toilet seat, steam room, sauna, jacuzzi, hot tub or pool.

SYMPTOMS

You can have NO SYMPTOMS or any of the following:

1. **Many exquisitely tender blister-like sores that appear 7 to 10 days after sex.** You may also have itching, tingling and/or burning before they actually appear and they typically last 7 to 14 days if this is your first infection.
2. **Pain when you urinate,** possibly urinating a lot, feeling like you can't hold it, urinating a little bit at a time or even not being able to urinate because your bladder is temporarily paralyzed.
3. **Swollen lymph nodes** in your inguinal skin folds just above each thigh.
4. Low-grade fever around **100.0 to 100.4F.**
5. **Fatigue.**
6. **One sore that comes and goes in the same place every few weeks or months** that is considerably less-painful and lasts only 2 to 4 days.

INFECTION COURSE

After your first genital herpes infection your sores eventually heal, but the HSV virus never dies. It quickly travels up your nerves and hides next to your spine. After 6 to 12 weeks your immune system starts making protective antibodies that help to keep your herpes hidden. You may already have some herpes antibodies if you already have periodic cold sores or fever blisters, but generally these do not fully protect you from a genital infection since there is usually 1one strain of herpes up top and another one below.

When your immune weakens however, HSV travels back down to the surface where it generally causes only a single sore since you now have antibodies around.

These antibodies also keep your newborn from getting herpes at birth if it comes in contact with one of these single sores.

If your immune system is too weak to make antibodies, you get many sores as if you had a first-time infection all over again.

DIAGNOSIS

Genital herpes is diagnosed if you have many painful sores 7 to 10 days after sex or a single less painful sore that comes and goes at the same place.

Sometimes a herpes tests is sent to confirm the diagnosis by roughly rubbing a Q-tip over your sore, then inserting it into a special room temperature gel or refrigerated viral culture solution that must be kept cold afterwards. Both are sent an outside lab for later analysis.

A negative result does not mean you do not have HSV however, because a sore can be contagious for as little as 48 hours if this is not your first infection. Not keeping the viral culture cold before and after transport to the lab can also affect your result.

Sometimes herpes is mentioned as an incidental finding on your PAP smear. In general, it does not pick up infections very well since it was designed to pick up pre-cancerous or cancerous changes on your cervix.

Blood tests for antibodies for HSV strains 1 AND 2 can be sent, but they are often inconclusive. As alluded to before, HSV-1 is found in mostly up top and HSV-2 is found mostly below. Some people have HSV-1 below and HSV-2 up top, however. Since most of you have had a cold sore or fever blister by early adolescence your blood test could already be positive for either HSV-1 or even HSV-2. This makes it hard to tell your positive result is from a new genital infection or an old cold sore or fever blister.

A lot of you look at me like I am stark raving mad when I tell you that you have a STD, yet you have not had sex for a while. I hate to burst your bubble, but mad I am not.

STD'S DO NOT GO AWAY JUST BECAUSE YOU STOP HAVING SEX!

You get STD's from sex, but the opposite is not true. STD's like genital herpes are more than happy to live inside you until you die—with or without sex—since your body supplies everything they need to survive!

TREATMENT

Herpes can be treated SUPPORTIVELY by:

1. Keeping your **skin clean and dry.**
2. **Not wearing** underwear, pantyhose or pants for a while.
3. **Taking over-the-counter (OTC) fever and pain medications** like Aspirin, Tylenol, Aleve, Advil, Nuprin or Motrin.
4. **Taking Prescribing Pyridium or OTC Uristat** if you have urinary symptoms.
5. **Having a sterile tube placed in your bladder** to drain it if it is temporarily paralyzed.
6. **Applying anesthetic ointments like prescription Lidocaine or OTC Vagicaine and Benzocaine** directly to particularly painful sores while you are waiting for anti-viral medication to work.

We prescribe ANTI-VIRAL medications if:

1. Your first infection is **particularly severe.**
2. **Your immune system is weak** from steroid medications, cancer treatment or HIV with or without AIDS.
3. **You have six or more infections a year.**
4. **You have a liver, brain or eye herpes infection** since these tend to be severe as well.

Herpes ANTI-VIRAL medications include:

1. **Acyclovir** / Zovirax 200mg tablets every 4 hours 5 times a day for 10 days that can be used with a 5% ointment if this is your first infection, 200mg every 4 hours 5 times a day for 5 days for other infections and 400mg twice daily if you have more than six or more infections a year.
2. **Valacyclovir** / Valtrex 1gram tablet twice daily for 10 days if this is your first infection, 500mg every 12 hours for 5 days for other infections and either 500mg twice daily if you have <9 infections a year or 1gram twice daily if you have >9 infections a year.
3. **Famciclovir** / Famvir 125mg tablet every 12 hours for 5 days for other infections and 250mg every 12 hours if you have 6 or more infections a year. It is not used for you first infection.

All can be used for severe infections during pregnancy.

Vasoline, OTC anti-fungals and anti-itch preparations like Vagisil, Vagi-Gard, Vaginex, Vagicaine, Benzocaine, Lanicaine, A+D, Summer's Eve Medicated, Gynecort, Hydrcortisone, Cortaid and Cortizone WILL NOT TREAT HERPES, only make it worse!

MALE INFECTION

Again, since genital herpes is a STD it would be criminal not to arm you with a little information about this infection in men!

Again, it primarily INFECTS their much longer penile urethra and SCROTUM or the wrinkled skin sac encasing the TESTICLES or balls.

Again, SYMPTOMS, DIAGNOSIS and TREATMENT are all the same.

Although barrier protection lowers your chances of infection, male condoms will not protect you from herpes that is not on or inside his penis!

20

Genital Warts

Genital warts—also called "Condyloma"—are included in the viral class of germ organisms since they are caused by an infection with Human Papilloma Virus or HPV.

Over 20 million Americans or 50% to 60% of sexually-active women have genital warts, myself included. Most are unaware of them however, since only 5% to 10% have been diagnosed! This is because HPV often lives in a quiet "turned off" state for weeks, months, years or decades when your immune system is able to control it. Obviously when your immune is unable to control it, HPV "turns on" and grows into warts. Even so, many warts are often missed because they are either too small to see and/or are located in concealed areas.

INFECTION SITES

While there are 70 different strains of HPV, only 15 of them infect your vulva, vagina, cervix, perineum, urethra, bladder, anus, rectum and buttocks.

CANCER SITES

There are 56 strains that are capable of causing cancer of your anus, vulva, vagina and cervix with 4 of these being strongly associated with the latter.

TRANSMISSION

HPV is the most common STD or SEXUALLY-TRANSMITTED DISEASE that is passed from person-to-person through close intimate sexual contact, including acts other than vaginal-penile penetration. This includes female-to-female sex as well as so-called virgins who engage in "heavy petting" without actually being penetrated!

TRANSLATION: He doesn't have to stick it in for you to get it! Just having his penis in the vicinity of your vulva and vaginal orifice is enough for you to get it!

It is important to remember that male condoms will not protect you from warts that are not on or inside his penis.

There is no way to know for sure who infected you nor when since HPV can live in a quiet "turned off" state for weeks, months, years or decades when your immune system is able to control it, before later growing into a genital wart. Again, the wart may have been there for a while, but too small for you to see and/or located in a concealed area.

You can also spread warts from your fingers to your genitals if you masturbate.

You can pass HPV to your newborn during birth as well and in 1 out of every 100,000 deliveries warts are found on a baby's vocal cords as a result of this. So many people have warts that some scientists suspect a lot more HPV is transferred at birth than we currently suspect.

In rare cases you can also get HPV from a warm soiled towel, underwear or bathing suit that has just been used by someone else, but if you do this you are probable having sex with that person. You can't get HPV from soiled towels, underwear or bathing suits that have been sitting around for a while, a moist toilet seat, steam room, sauna, jacuzzi, hot tub or pool.

DIAGNOSIS

Genital warts are easy to diagnose if you have CAULIFLOWER GROWTHS.

If your growth does not have this typical appearance, A TISSUE BIOPSY may be needed in the office under local anesthesia at a cost of $100 to $300.

Since cervical warts are generally too small to see, most are picked up by PAP smears, which cost only $24 to $40 and are discussed in detailed in the next chapter.

The remainder are picked up by the DIGENE HYBRID CAPTURE HPV-DNA test that is sent right after your PAP by swabbing your cervix with a Q-tip, brush or broom from the special ThinPrep PAP kit or sending your tissue biopsy in a special transport solution.

The FDA just approved a less expensive $40 to $50 HIGH-RISK VERSION of this test that specifically looks for HPV strains associated with cervical cancer, including the particularly aggressive16 and 18 strains.

A lot of you look at me like I am stark raving mad when I tell you that you have a STD, yet you have not had sex for a while. I hate to burst your bubble, but mad I am not.

STD'S DO NOT GO AWAY JUST BECAUSE YOU STOP HAVING SEX!

You get STD's from sex, but the opposite is not true. STD's like genital warts are more than happy to live inside you until you die—with or without sex—since your body supplies everything they need to survive!

TREATMENT

While genital warts can be treated, they are rarely cured! This is because it is almost impossible to detect "turned off" HPV that is lurking under the surface that can "turn on" and grow later on! Additionally, you can pick up new HPV strains from future partners since so many people are infected.

Several treatments are listed below, but none is better than the others.

1. **Aldara / Imiquimod 5% cream** is applied to the skin adjacent to your warts three times a week up to 4 months until they disappear. It stimulates the natural immune boosters in your skin that combat HPV growth.
2. **Condylox / Podofilox 0.5% solution and/or gel** is applied twice daily for 3 days, followed by 4 days of rest and repeating this 3-day on and 4-day off cycle three more times until they disappear. This destroys your wart, its underlying and adjacent skin surfaces.
3. **Podphyllin Resin 10 to 15%** is more potent so it is applied weekly in the office. You must wash it off 6 hours later or you will get a severe chemical burn!
4. **TCA or BCA / Tri-chloroacetic or Bi-chloroacetic acid 80 to 90%** is also applied in the office every 5 to 7 days up to 4 applications. It tingles and burns for the first 5 to 10 minutes and also destroys your wart, its underlying and adjacent skin surfaces. This is the only topical method used in pregnancy.
5. **Efudex / Fluorouracil 2% cream** aggressively destroys all surfaces it comes into contact with so frequent office visits are

required to carefully monitor its resultant inflammation and scarring. A Q-tip is used to apply it thrice weekly if your warts are around your urethral meatus. It is also applied to a tampon that you insert and leave inside your vagina for 20 minutes also thrice weekly if you have warts there. You must take a bath afterwards however, to wash away any leftover cream.

6. **Rarely, Alferon N / Interferon alfa-n3 can be injected** into the base of warts that are particularly persistent twice daily up to 8 weeks. It causes flu-like side effects however, that are quite unpleasant.
7. **Cryotherapy or freezing therapy** in the office can be used if you have cervical warts and also if you have a few relatively small warts on your vulva and/or in your vagina.
8. **Infrared Coagulator (IRC) or infrared light burn therapy** is also used in the office if you have a few relatively small warts on your vulva and/or just inside your vagina. This done after applying a local anesthetic ointment then an injection.
9. **Electrocautery or electrical burn therapy** is used for vulva warts as well. This is performed in the office under local anesthesia if you have a few small ones OR in an outpatient surgery center while under deeper anesthesia if you have a lot. Since your exposed raw skin takes several weeks to heal, your warts are burned off a little at a time several weeks apart if they cover a large area.
10. **Laser or intensive light burn therapy** under anesthesia in an outpatient surgery center is also used if you have warts on your cervix, in your vagina and/or if you have a lot of vulva warts. Again, it takes several weeks for you to heal so they are burned off a little at a time if you they cover a large area.
11. **Surgical excision via a scalpel knife or Loop Electrocurrent Electrocautery Procedure (LEEP) using an electrified thin loop of wire** can be performed in the office under local under anesthesia if

you have a few small vulva and/or vaginal warts OR in an outpatient surgical center while under deeper anesthesia if you have a few particularly large vulva and/or vaginal warts.

12. **If you are pregnant, we only remove large warts that block your vaginal orifice one to two months before your expected delivery.** This is because warts tend to worsen as your pregnancy progresses and they are likely to come back if they are removed too early. Premature labor and early delivery are possible risks as well.

Not smoking, rest, sleep, good diet and avoiding stress are just as important in strengthening your immune system and its ability to control HPV.

50% to 60% of microscopic warts and 15% to 20% of visible ones "turn off" within 3 to 6 months if your immune system has the ability to control them.

Therefore, if you have HIV, it is important for you to monitor it and treat it as aggressively as you can.

If you are using steroid creams like Lidex and Hydrocortisone, try to stop them if you can since they weaken your immune system as well.

You should continue steroid asthma inhalers and Prednisone tablet therapy, however.

Of course, you should also continue any life-saving cancer treatments, even if they weaken your immune system.

MALE INFECTION

Again, since genital warts are a STD it would be criminal not to arm you with a little information about this infection in men!

HPV primarily infects their penile urethra and SCROTUM or the wrinkled skin sac encasing their TESTICLES or balls.

HPV additionally causes cancer of the penis.

Again, DIAGNOSIS is easy if you have cauliflower growths!

Since warts in males are often hidden down inside the penile urethra or bladder, however:

1. **He should see a dermatologist, urologist or even your gynecological medical professional for an ANDROSCOPY exam of his outer genitals.** First a dilute vinegar solution is applied to make warts show up better, then the entire outer genital area is meticulously scanned using an extremely bright light and a magnifying device. This requires a considerable amount of time since there is a lot more skin to cover, particularly the all the folds that make up the wrinkled scrotum. As a result, it generally costs hundreds of dollars.
2. **Next, his urine should be checked for blood even if no warts are seen on the outer genitals. If blood is detected, he should be referred to an Urologist for a CYSTOSCOPY.** This surgery introduces a telescope into the penile urethra and bladder under anesthesia to look for warts and costs hundreds of dollars as well. The risk of this procedure includes infection, perforation injury if the telescope punctures the urethra and/or bladder and stricture if excess scar tissue forms and blocks urine flow.
3. **Given the expense and risks associated with cystoscopy, he may want to consider one of the Digene Hybrid Capture HPV-DNA testing of his penile urethra first to see if it is really needed.** Your gynecological medical professional will have to perform this testing since it is approved for use only in women and most Urologists are not familiar with it.

Again, TISSUE BIOPSY may be performed on any growths that are seen.

Again, TREATMENT is the same.

Although barrier protection lowers your chances of infection, male condoms will not protect you from warts that are not on or inside his penis!

By the way, if HPV was diagnosed while you are currently being intimate with someone, protection may be of little or no use since both of you are probably sharing the same HPV strains already.

21

PAP Smear

Finally, this book ends with the anxiety-laden PAP smear test, which picks up PRE-CANCEROUS AND CANCEROUS CERVICAL CHANGES that sometimes appear after your cervix has been infected with HPV or Human Papilloma Virus (see prior chapter). Pre-cancerous changes occur before cervical cancer actually develops months, years or decades later and HPV is the virus that causes genital warts, the most common STD or Sexually-Transmitted Disease that is passed from person-to-person during sex.

The PAP is a cheap preliminary screening test that is cheap and easy to perform as opposed to the more expensive and involved diagnostic testing that may be required if your results are not normal. This means that the PAP is less accurate, but it only costs $24 to $40 and can be done by a non-Gynecological medical professional in one quick office, clinic or ER visit. In contrast, the more accurate diagnostic tests cost hundreds to thousands of dollars and require several specialty Gynecology office or clinic visits.

Do not panic if your PAP result is not normal since pre-cancer is found in only 10% to 20% and actual cervical cancer itself is an extremely rare finding! In the US in 1999, there were only 12,800 new cases of cervical cancer, which accounted for only 2% of all new cancer cases in women, and only 4,800 deaths from it.

Since the PAP was not designed to pick up other infections, it does this poorly! Therefore, it should never be substituted for Gonorrhea, Chlamydia and Herpes testing or a Saline Prep test of your vaginal discharge whenever Yeast, Trichomonas, Bacterial Vaginosis and/or DIV (see these chapters) are suspected.

TECHNIQUE

For those of you who wondered how the PAP is done, wonder no more.

1. **First we gently introduce a speculum** into your vagina to reach your cervix.
2. **The outer portion of your cervix is scraped with a wooden stick** that is smeared onto both sides of a glass slide labeled with your name.
3. **A wire-bristle brush or Q-tip is then twirled inside your cervical canal** and smeared onto the other half of the same slide. You may have some bleeding after this, especially if you have an infection.
4. **Next, your slide is sprayed with a solution that preserves** anywhere from 50,000 to 300,000 cells.
5. **Then it is sent to an outside lab with a form** that has your name, age, date of your last period, whether or not your cervix is irritated, if you had any recent pelvic surgeries and other PAP's that were not normal.
6. **Specially trained lab technicians scan your slide under a microscope** after it is submerged in dyes that make these 50,000 to 300,000 cells show up better.

7. **The technician gives your slide a result that is confirmed by a doctor.**
8. **Many large labs also have automated machines to check your results as well.** This added feature almost doubles the cost of your PAP test.
9. **Your results are returned within 5 to 14 days** in the form of a printed report.
10. **The ThinPrep PAP technique is a little different since it provides a broom-like device that is used to scrape your outer and inner cervix. Then it is placed in a vial of preservative fluid.** This vial is sent to the lab where your cervical cells are separated from any interfering discharge, blood and mucus. Your cervical cells are smeared onto a slide that is also scanned. This special PAP costs about $45 to $60 though.

INDICATIONS

You should have a PAP:

1. **Once you start having sex and are exposed to HPV.**
2. **Every year** if your last PAP was normal.
3. **Every year even if you had a total hysterectomy** or surgical removal of your uterus and its cervix since a tiny portion of it can always be left behind unintentionally. A VAGINAL PAP is sent after scraping the cells from the back of your vagina with the wooden stick.
4. **Every 6 months if you have HIV** even if the PAP was normal because your immune system is weak and less able to fight off HPV.
5. **Every 3 months** if the last PAP was not normal.
6. **Every 3 years** if 3 prior yearly PAP's were all normal.

7. **You do not need a PAP if you are a virgin or lesbian** who has never been penetrated by a penis, tongue, finger, vibrators or dildo.

WAYS TO IMPROVE ACCURACY

You can have a PAP anytime, but your results will be more accurate if:

1. **Your 50,000 to 300,000 cervical cells are not covered with interfering blood, sperm and semen after recent sex, vaginal suppositories and creams, amniotic fluid and mucus during labor.** The ThinPrep PAP does this quite well since it separates your cervical cells from any interfering discharge, blood and mucus before they are smeared onto a slide.
2. **You do not have a cervical infection since the discharge** from it contains interfering infecting organisms and inflammatory white cells that similarly cover your 50,00 to 300,000 cervical cells while also creating confusing changes that resemble precancer.
3. **You do not douche and wash away your cervical cells.** This actually gives you infections and never cleans you so it is not recommended for routine hygiene, odor and/or increased discharge!
4. **You wait 3 to 4 months for your cervical cells to grow back** after they are removed by a prior PAP, Gonorrhea and/or Chlamydia test, miscarriage, abortion, vaginal delivery, Cesarean section and surgeries involving your cervix.

REPORT REQUIREMENTS

Your PAP report must mention whether or not your specimen was ADEQUATE or containing inner cells as well as outer ones. It will be INADEQUATE and only 50% complete if inner cells are missing. If you have undergone a total hysterectomy with removal of your cervix as well as your uterus, only vaginal cells are expected, however.

Your PAP report may also mention whether or not it was SATISFACTORY or if both sets of cells were clearly seen. It will be UNSATISFACTORY if you have a lot of discharge, blood, semen or medication in your vagina that covers up your 50,000 to 300,000 cervical cells.

REPORT RESULTS

Your PAP report may mention if you have any germ organisms like Yeast fungus, Trichomonas parasite, Herpes virus, Lactobacilli and Coccobacilli bacteria. Again, it does this poorly since it misses far more of these infections than it picks up! Also, this does not mean that you really have an infection since yeast and certain bacteria normally live in your vagina.

Your PAP report must mention what your cervical cells looked like (or your vaginal cells if you had a total hysterectomy). Typical results are listed below.

1. **NORMAL or NEGATIVE.**
2. **INFLAMMATORY CHANGES** from an identified infection or an unidentified one that usually requires an office saline prep microscopic discharge exam as well as sampling for later Gonorrhea and/or Chlamydia lab testing.
3. **ASCUS or Atypical Squamous Cells of Undetermined Significance.**

    "Atypical" means not typical, but not pre-cancer or cancer. **"Squamous"** is the type of cell that comes from your outer cervix. **"Undetermined Significance"** means that the lab cannot determine if your abnormal cells are due to an infection, a hidden pre-cancer that is later found in 10 to 20% or a hidden cancer that is later found in 0.1%.

Unfortunately, 50% of cervical cancer patients had ACSUS on their last PAP.

4. **AGCUS or Atypical Glandular Cells of Undetermined Significance** is similar to **ASCUS** with "Glandular" being the type of cell that comes from your inner cervical canal.
5. **HPV CHANGES that occur early in your HPV infection** before pre-cancer has a chance to develop.
6. **PRE-CANCER, DYSPLASIA, CIN OR SIL are all the same.**

   DYSPLASIA means "abnormal growth" in Latin and is categorized as **MILD, MODERATE or SEVERE.**

   CIN stands for "Cervical Intraepithelial Neoplasia" and is categorized as **CIN1, CIN2 and CIN3, also called CIS** or Carcinoma in Situ in some labs.

   SIL stands for "Squamous Intraepitheial Lesion" and is categorized as Low-Grade (**LGSIL** or Lo-SIL), which is CIN1 or High-Grade (**HGSIL** or Hi-SIL), which includes both CIN2 and CIN3.
7. **CANCER** that is further categorized as being **SUSPICIOUS or POSITIVE.**

Your PAP may also mention what your endometrial cells looked like if you were bleeding. These cells were shed from the lining of your upper uterine cavity and are categorized as being **NORMAL or ABNORMAL.**

MANGEMENT

If your PAP was inadequate, unsatisfactory or inflammatory, it is repeated 3 to 4 months after treating any infections identified during your exam or on a subsequent saline prep during a visit afterwards.

If your PAP was ASCUS, it is also repeated 3 to 4 months later, preferably after treating any infections.

If there is no infection to treat, a HPV-DNA TEST should be considered to look for the thirteen strains associated with cervical cancer, particularly the aggressive 16 and 18 strains. The Digene High-Risk Hybrid Capture HPV-DNA Q-tip or brush test (see prior chapter) costs about $40 to $50. If it is positive, you should then have a colposcopy as explained below.

If you do not want to wait however, COLPOSCOPY can be done to carefully scan your outer cervix and the opening of its inner canal with a magnifying device over 10 to 30 minutes. This is strongly recommended if you already have genital warts and/or HIV. If you have any areas that look like HGSIL and/or cancer, they are biopsied in the office and sent to an outside lab for a more definite tissue diagnosis. This is called CXBX or cervical biopsy. Most of the time, the remaining inner cells that cannot be seen are scraped off and sent to an outside lab as well. This is called ECC or endocervical curettage. Either result takes 2 to 3 working days.

Since colposcopy costs $200 to $400, repeating the PAP is a cheap alternative while you put money aside for one. This is reasonable since ASCUS generally improves over time, especially if it was caused by an infection. Also, only 10 to 20% of those with ASCUS have hidden pre-cancer and only 0.1% hidden cancer.

If your PAP was AGCUS, you can opt for an ECC prior to repeating the PAP in 10 to 12 weeks after treating any identifiable infections. Again, this generally improves if it was due to an identifiable infection. Since underlying pre-cancer or cancer can be present however, you may also want to consider a Digene High-Risk Hybrid Capture HPV-DNA Q-tip test and/or colposcopy just in case your outer cervix has other abnormalities that were missed.

If your PAP was HPV CHANGES and/or LGSIL, it is repeated 3 to 4 months later or a colposcopy is done instead. Both HPV changes and LGSIL can improve over time if your immune system is strong and if you do not have aggressive 16 and/or 18 HPV strains. Generally, it takes years for either to progress to HGSIL and/or cancer, though 15 to 25 % of those with LGSIL actually have HGSIL that is hidden.

If your PAP was HGSIL, you need a colposcopy and ECC as well as a possible CXBX from any areas of your cervix that appear suggestive.

If your PAP was cancer, you need a CXBX with or without colposcopy. Usually, the cancer is obvious though colposcopy will reveal it if not.

If your PAP had abnormal endometrial cells, an EMBX or endometrial biopsy should be done. This result also takes 2 to 3 working days.

SURGICAL TREATMENT

You may end up having any of the surgical treatments below as well.

1. **CRYOTHERAPY freezes** your cervix in the office if you have persistent ASCUS, AGCUS, HPV changes or LGSIL.
2. **LEEP or Loop Electrocurrent Electrocautery Procedure uses an electrified loop of thin wire** to cut out portions of your cervix in the office under local anesthesia if you have LGSIL and CIN2-HGSIL that does not involve your canal. This tissue is sent to the lab with the results taking 2 to 3 working days.
3. **CONE BIOPSY removes an ice cream cone-like portion your cervix** in the hospital under deeper anesthesia to treat LGSIL and CIN2 that involves your canal, CIN2+CIN3-HGSIL and PAP-biopsy discrepancies where your result is a lot worse that your CXBX and/or ECC that may have missed your abnormal area. Again, this tissue is sent to the lab with the results taking 2 to 3 working days.
4. **Cervical cancer requires a lot of other tests to see if it has spread.** Early cervical cancer is sometimes treated with cone biopsy or total hysterectomy. More advanced cervical cancer requires radiation and sometimes even chemotherapy.

MORE PEARLS OF WISDOM

Do not "shop around" for the result you want by immediately running off to another office or clinic to have your PAP repeated without waiting 10 to 12 weeks for your cervical cells to grow back and without letting them know the results of your prior abnormal PAP.

Again, wait 10 to 12 weeks before repeating your PAP if it has inflammatory changes, ASCUS, AGCUS, HPV changes or LGSIL.

Again, arrange for an immediate colposcopy if your PAP has HGSIL or cancer.

SINCE HGSIL AND/OR CANCER NEVER DISAPPEARS INTO THIN AIR, be very suspicious of a normal/negative, inflammatory changes, HPV changes, ASCUS or LGSIL result if you choose to repeat your PAP without a colposcopy!

References

Altman A, Endocrine Issues In Special Populations Lecture, *Critical Endocrine Issues In Women Conference* sponsored by the Joslin Diabtes Center, February 2000.

Ashley-Gilbert A, Barker B, Broekhuizen F, Verga C, Advances in Managing Genital Warts, *Supplement to OBG Management*, June 2000.

Barakat R, Contemporary Issues in the Management of Endometrial Cancer, *CA-A Cancer Journal for Clinicians*, 48:5, 1998.

Beck W, Management of Atypical and Low-Grade Squamous Intraepithelial Pap Smears, *Postgraduate Obstetrics & Gynecology*, 18:6, 1998.

Bazil C, Optimal Use of Anitepileptic Drugs, *Merritt-Putnam Lectures on Epilepsy* Conference sponsored by the Columbia-Presbyterian and Montfiore Medical Centers, September 2000.

Broditsky R, Fitzpatrick L, Notelovitz M, Sharma S, Utian W, HRT and Heart Health: What the Experts are Doing Now, *OBG Management*, 12:6, 2000.

Campion M, Greenberg M, Turner F, New Horizons in Cervical Cancer Screening, *ACOG Monograph*, 1996.

Carter J, Combined Hysteroscopic and Laparoscopic Findings in Patients with Chronic Pelvic Pain, *J Am Association of Gynecological Laparoscopists*, 2(1): 43-47, 1994.

Centers for Disease Control and Prevention, 1998 Guidelines for Treatment of Sexually-Transmitted Diseases, *MMWR 1998*, 47:RR-1.

Comp P, Coagulation and Thrombosis with OC Use: Physiology and Clinical Relevance, *Dialogues in Contraception*, 5:1, 1996.

Darney P, Klaisle C, Contraception-Associated Menstrual Problems: Etiology and Management, *Dialogues in Contraception*, 5:5, 1998.

Fauci A, Braunwald E, Isselbacher K, Wilson J, Martin J, Kasper D, Hauser S, Longo D, *Harrison's Principles of Internal Medicine, McGraw-Hill, 1998.*

Gromes D, Chaney E, Connell E, Creinin M, Emans S, Goldzieher J, Hillard P, Mastroianni L, Specially-Packaged Emergency Contraception Comes to US, *The Contraception Report*, 9:6, 1999.

Gromes D, Chaney E, Connell E, Creinin M, Emans S, Goldzieher J, Hillard P, Mastroianni L, Levonorgestrel Alone for Emergency Contraception, *The Contraception Report*, 9:6, 1999.

Heller R, Heller R, Vagnini F, *The Carbohydrate Addict's Healthy Heart Program*, Ballantine Books, 1999.

Hudson T, *Women's Encyclopedia of Natural Medicine*, Keats Publishing, 1999.

Kanuitz A, Medroxyprogesterone Acetate / Estradiol Cypionate: Overview of a new Contraceptive, *Dialogues in Contraception*, 6:1, 1999.

Kurman J, *Blaustein's Pathology of the Female Genital Tract*, 3rd ed., Springer-Verlag, New York, 1987.

Landis S, Murray T, Bolden S, Wingo P, Cancer Statistics, 1998, *CA-A Cancer Journal for Clinicians*, 48:1, 1998.

Love S, Lindsey K, *Dr. Susan Love's Hormone Book*, Times Books, 1998.

Mishell D, Kaunitz A, Sulak P, Westhoff C, Oral Contraceptives and Venous Thromboembolism Consensus Conference Statement, *Dialogues in Contraception*, 1996.

Mishell D, Speroff L, Grimes P, Westhoff C, Kaunitz A, Pasquale S, Burkman R, Intrauterine Contraception in the U. S., *University of Minnesota Conference Proceedings Monograph*, Health Learning Systems, 1996.

Mishell D, Mattox J, Shulman L, Bush T, Arias R, Lifetime Hormonal Management Lecture Series, *Video Satellite Conference* sponsored by PremEdCo, Inc., January 2000.

Mishell D, Sulak P, The IUD: Dispelling the Myths and Assessing the Potential, *Dialogues in Contraception*, 5:5, 1997.

Northrup C, *Women's Bodies, Women's Wisdom*, revised edition, Bantam Books, 1998.

Rosenberg R, A Physiological Approach to Managing PMDD Lecture, *Depression and PMDD Conference* sponsored by CME, Inc. in conjunction with CMEA, Inc., May 2000.

Rosenfeld J, Alley N, Acheson L, Admire J, *Women's Health in Primary Care*, Williams & Wilkins, 1977.

Scialli A, Evaluating the Patient with Chronic Pelvic Pain, *Supplement to OBG Management*, February 2000.

Speroff L, Glass R, Kase N, *Clinical Gynecologic Endocrinology and Infertility*, 6th ed, Lippincott Williams & Wilkins, 1999.

Sulak P, Kaunitz A, Hormonal Contraception and Bone Mineral Density, *Dialogues in Contraception*, 6:2, 1999.

Westhoff C, A Perspective on the Concept of Risk, *Dialogues in Contraception*, 5:1, 1996.

On-line Sources:

The Aeron LifeCycles Laboratory, http://www.aeron.com.

The American Heart Association, http://www.americanheart.org/statistics/biostats/biowo.htm.

The American Cancer Society, *http://www.cancer.org/statistics/index.html.*

The Cytyc Corporation, *http://www.cytyc.com*.

The Digene Corporation, *http://www.digene.com*.

The Food and Drug Administration, http://www.fda.gov.

The National Osteoporosis Foundation, http://nof.org/osteoporosis/stats.htm.

Index

A

C

E

F

G

H

treatment, 22, 32, 53-54, 56, 62, 64, 67-68, 74, 85, 91-93, 98, 100, 104, 106, 114, 117, 121-123, 126, 129, 134, 139, 141-142, 147, 149-150, 156, 161-162, 168-169, 173, 176, 185, 188

urethritis, 125, 149, 158-162

I

L

M

O

P

S

T

V

X

Y